Keto Diet and Intermittent Fasting for Women

This Book Includes:

The Ultimate Guide to Mastering Healthy Weight Loss with Ketogenic and IF Lifestyle. Includes a 30-Day Meal Plan with Tasty Keto Recipes.

D1607560

by

Dorothy Smith PhD

Table of Contents

Keto Diet for Women

Intermittent Fasting for Women

Keto Diet for Women

The Ultimate Guide to Mastering Healthy Weight Loss with Ketogenic Lifestyle. Includes a 30-Day Meal Plan with Tasty Keto Recipes to Promote Longevity & Boost Your Energy.

by

Dorothy Smith PhD

Part One: Getting Started

Chapter 1: Keto Diet Explained

There are many diets gaining traction today, but none like the ketogenic diet. However, the interesting thing about this diet is that it is not used for weight loss. For the past century, it has been used as a way to treat epilepsy. However, because this diet is so temperamental, this is only done with the strictest doctor supervision. The ketogenic diet is a diet that is designed to release ketones in your bloodstream. Many of the cells in your body prefer to use blood sugar, which it gets from carbohydrates, as your body's main source of energy. The idea of the ketogenic diet is to put your body in a state of ketosis. This means the absence of circulating blood sugar from food and your body breaking down stored fat into the molecules called ketone bodies. When you reach ketosis, it is believed that more of your cells will use the ketone bodies for generating energy until you eat carbs again. This varies between person to person, so you need to be careful.

A warning that this book will give you before we proceed is that the ketogenic diet is not considered to be safe. Doctors all over the world and from the most prestigious medical practices advise against it for a few reasons. The first being that this diet was only invented to help people in the most extreme situations and even then not forever. Doctors recommend this diet for no longer than six months and even then only under constant contact and supervision by a doctor that you see. It has also been shown to put certain people into a state called ketoacidosis, which can be fatal. This is especially true in diabetics. They could die in under an hour. It can also worsen those with kidney disease as well as making you have sleep problems and stomach issues along with constipation and vomiting. Another downside is this diet has been shown to be heavy on red meat and other processed foods that are salty and fatty, which is unhealthy. You should also avoid keto if your pregnant as it could harm your unborn child as well as yourself.

That being said, the ketogenic diet is a diet that lacks carbohydrates and concentrates on proteins and fats. There are four different types of ketogenic diets, and you should be aware of all four as they differ in certain aspects. The first diet is the targeted diet. This will allow you to eat carbs, but you can only do so around workouts.

The next is the high protein diet. This one is similar to the basic diet, but obviously, it will include more protein. The numbers that this diet offers is 5% carbs, 35% protein, and 60% fat.

The third is the cyclical diet. This diet involves what is known as refeeding. The basis for this diet is that you have periods of higher-carb refeeds. For example, you have five ketogenic diet days and then two high carb days.

The last diet is the basic diet. This is the one that is used most often and by most people. The numbers for this one are as follows, 75% fat with only 5% carbs and 20% protein.

It is worth noting that the only two diets that have been studied extensively are the basic and high protein diet. The other two are more advanced, and bodybuilders and athletes are the ones that generally use them, although it's not ideal or recommended since they need further study.

The ketogenic diet believes that it is an effective way to lose weight and help lower your risk factors for disease. It is also believed to be filling, and you can lose weight without having to count your calories or track what you're eating. However, this isn't true. The ketogenic diet makes you track your food very carefully because you need to know where your fat and carbs are, as well as the protein content. If you're not tracking these things, you could throw yourself out of where you are supposed to be.

Another benefit is that it is believed that it can help with diabetes. This is because it can help you lose excess fat, which is very closely related to diabetes. Especially type 2 diabetes. One study found that it can improve insulin sensitivity by 75%. However, this should be looked into more as other studies have found problems with this diet. Another belief is that it can help with cancer, Alzheimer's disease, and heart disease.

We have already mentioned that it has been used to treat epilepsy, but it is also said that it can help with polycystic ovary syndrome or PCS for short as well as Parkinson's disease. Brain injuries have been studied in one animal study, but there is much more research that is needed to be conclusive. On the lower scale, it may be able to help with acne as well.

Why is the keto diet so effective for weight loss? If you don't consume enough carbs from your food; your cells will begin to burn fat for the necessary energy instead. Your body will switch over to ketosis for its energy source as you cut back on carbs and calories.

Two elements that occur when your body doesn't need the glucose:

The Stage of Lipogenesis: If there is a sufficient supply of glycogen in your liver and muscles, any excess is converted to fat and stored.

The Stage of Glycogenesis: The excess of glucose converts to glycogen and is stored in the muscles and liver. Research indicates that only about half of your energy used daily can be saved as glycogen.

Your body will have no more food (similar to when you are sleeping) making your body burn the fat to create ketones. Once the ketones break down the fats, which generate fatty acids, they will burn-off in the liver through beta-oxidation. Thus, when you no longer have a supply of glycogen or glucose, ketosis begins and will use the consumed/stored fat as energy.

The keto diet will set up your body to deplete the stored glucose. Once that is accomplished, your body will focus on diminishing the stored fat you have saved as fuel. Many people don't understand that counting calories don't matter at this point since it is just used as a baseline. Your body doesn't need glucose which will trigger these two stages:

The State of Glycogenesis: The excess of glucose converts itself into glycogen which is stored in the muscles and liver. Research indicates only about <u>half</u> of your energy used daily can be saved as glycogen.

The State of Lipogenesis: This phase is introduced when there is an adequate supply of glycogen in your liver and muscles, with any excess being converted to fat and stored.

Your body will have no more food (similar to the times when you are sleeping) making your body burn the fat to create ketones. Once the ketones break down the fats, which generate fatty acids, they will burn-off in the liver through beta-oxidation. Thus, when you no longer have a supply of glycogen or glucose, ketosis begins and will use the consumed/stored fat as energy.

When the glycerol and fatty acid molecules are released, the ketogenesis process begins, and acetoacetate is produced. The Acetoacetate is converted to two types of ketone units:

Acetone: This is mostly excreted as waste but can also be metabolized into glucose. This is the reason individuals on a ketogenic diet will experience a distinctive smelly breath.

Beta-hydroxybutyrate or BHB: Your muscles will convert the acetoacetate into BHB which will fuel your brain after you have been on the keto diet for a short time.

There are many foods that you can eat on this diet, but there are many foods that you can't, and its this subject, in particular, that we're going to go into now. The following foods that you need to avoid eating are the following.

- Fruit- You will need to avoid all fruits except small portions of certain kinds like berries.
- Beans- Peas and beans like kidney beans are to be avoided as well because they are too high in carbs.
- Legumes- Lentils will also need to be avoided.
- Starches and grains -Wheat products like pasta and cereal are a big no-no, and you will have to stay away from these as well.
- Sugary foods- fruit juice, smoothies, junk food, and things like ice cream and cake are out as well.
- sugar -free foods-These are most often found in sugar alcohols or diet foods that claim to help you lose weight. They are very highly processed, and they can affect your ketone levels in a negative way.

- Alcohol-The carb content on these is very high, and they can knock you out of where you need to be.
- Root vegetables or tubers-This category means potatoes (including sweet potatoes) and things like carrots.
- Unhealthy fats-You should seriously limit your intake of the fats that are processed. This includes mayonnaise and vegetable oil.
- Diet items and low-fat items-These are overloaded with carbs and are extremely processed.
- Condiments and sauces- They contain too much sugar and fat that is unhealthy.

The foods that you should eat on this diet to make sure that you are following it correctly are the following. As we have stated above, some of these foods are unhealthy such as forms of coconut oil and red meats.

- Healthy oils-The three main ones to focus on are avocado oil, extra virgin olive oil, and coconut oil.

- Cheese-You can eat many different varieties, such as mozzarella, cheddar, cream, or blue. You should go for unprocessed cheeses.
- Eggs-Look for omega-3 whole eggs or pastured eggs.
- Fatty fish-Salmon, tuna, mackerel, and trout are all good options for you.
- Meat-Turkey, bacon, chicken, and sausage are all good options. Red meat and steak are other options as well.
- Butter-Try and get grass-fed if you can.
- Cream- As with butter, if you can find grass-fed, then go for that.
- Nuts-Almonds and walnuts are great options here.
- Seeds-Pumpkin seeds, flax seeds, and chia seeds are all good options, but a warning is that many seeds can cause issues with your digestion and stomach.
- Low carb vegetables-Most green vegetables are alright, and you can have peppers, onions, and tomatoes as well.
- Avocados-You can use them for guacamole, or you can eat them whole. Whole avocados can be used for so many recipes.

- Spices-You can use herbs and spices (healthy ones) and salt and pepper in moderation, of course.

Other healthy foods that you can eat as long as you are careful because the numbers vary as far as carbs (though most are zero and others go as high as 7 grams).

- Lamb
- Jerky
- Veal
- Bison
- Venison
- Sardines
- Shellfish (careful on this one the carbs will add up)
- Catfish
- Cod
- Herring
- Lobster
- Haddock
- Broccoli
- Cauliflower
- Brussels sprouts

- Kale
- Eggplant
- Asparagus
- Cucumber
- Mushrooms
- Green beans
- Celery
- Spinach
- Cabbage
- Swiss chard
- Zucchini
- Olives
- Strawberries
- Grapefruit (be careful on this one the carbs can get really high very quickly)
- Apricots
- Lemons
- Kiwis
- Mulberries
- Oranges
- Raspberries
- Peanuts
- Sunflower seeds
- Pistachios
- Macadamia nuts

- Hazelnuts
- Cashews
- Coconuts
- Full fat yogurt
- Greek yogurt
- Lard
- Tallow
- Coffee
- Tea
- Carbonated water
- Club soda
- Dark chocolate (choose a real dark chocolate with 70 percent cocoa at least)

Food is such an important part of this diet that it's important to make sure that you're informed on it so that you can have the best knowledge and the knowledge that is going to be of the most useful to you. Having the right information means you can be successful; having the wrong information can lead to injuries or worse. Doctors have said that you should always ask them before starting this diet at all, but this is proven to be more true if you have the following health issues.

- Obesity
- Heart conditions
- High blood pressure
- Diabetes
- Kidney issues
- Cancer
- Epilepsy

The reason that you should have their supervision is because these are all serious conditions. Especially things like cancer and epilepsy.

Exercise is so important on this diet as well, and it is important to understand how you need to utilize it for your benefit. Exercise is important in any diet that you choose, and it's important to be able to understand that exercise is what you need to become a healthier person, but it can actually be harder on the keto diet because your body is being put through so much already.

As such, your routine is going to change. The main reason is because your not using carbs for energy and fuel, your using fat for fuel. Fat doesn't give you that energy burst that you need for push-ups or jumps like carbs do. You will probably not feel like working out at all because of how your feelings, but you will be able to get past this, and you will be able to make a good routine for yourself.

Because workouts like sprinting, weightlifting, and high-intensity interval training are workouts all require that quick burst of energy, they are going to be much more strenuous though many say it won't be impossible. Just remember the reason for this is because the fat in your body is not as available to your muscles as the energy that you get from carbs are. Because of this, you are more likely to get tired during these workouts and much quicker than you usually do.

This doesn't mean you have to stop working out; it means you have to be smarter about how you work out. Jogging and bike riding are both great options for you to do on this diet, and a good rule of thumb is to go for something that is low to moderate as far as your workout and do something for a short duration. This is especially true for the first two weeks that you start this. With your doctor's permission, you can talk to them about going into higher amounts of workout, but you need to have their help with this, so check with them first.

If your feeling drained on the basic diet, another option is to try the targeted diet or the cyclical diet. This is not recommended for a lot of people, so this would be another area where you need to check with your doctor as well to see if this is alright for you. Another issue with doing this is that you will knock yourself out of that ketosis state that they want you to stay in. Overall, it has been proven that working out doesn't feel as good on the keto diet as it did before. This is another reason that the keto diet isn't for everyone. If you love exercising, this isn't the best choice for you. This is especially true because exercise is important for health.

It is recommended that along with speaking to your doctor about what exercises are good for you to do for yourself, is to speak to a nutritionist professional and a certified trainer as well. This will make sure that you have a great workout plan that is safe. You should also not do any workouts that you haven't done before. This is because this diet can affect how that workout is going to affect you, and the result could be very negative. Other tips that you need to be aware of is that when your working out on this diet are the following tips.

Listen to your body and what it's telling you. You should never keep going or pushing if your body is telling you it can't do it or handle it. If your body is telling you to stop, then you need to stop. Feelings of dizziness and exhaustion or even just fatigue are all signs that you should stop. They are not normal, and this is a sign that your body isn't responding well to this diet and that you need a doctor's help.

Make sure that you are eating enough. This is another big thing with this diet, and this doesn't just include keeping your calorie count where it needs to be. This means keeping your fat where it needs to be, as well. Remember that when your exercising, your body normally uses carbs then fat. Now your using fat. So if you're not taking in enough nutrition, you are not going to be able to handle even the simplest workout. You could actually be putting yourself in danger.

Avoid high-intensity workouts. This is so important with the keto diet. More is not better. In many cases, this is something that is true. The keto diet is considered to be an extreme diet, and as such, you won't be able to do what you are normally able to do. You have to be able to understand that high-intensity workouts are something that is no longer going to be able for you to do. Instead, remember that you really need to stick to a lower intensity workout instead. This is really important particularly important when your starting this diet and for at least the first month that you're doing this.

This diet puts a lot of stress on your body, and it can take a very long time to adjust if your actually able to adjust at all. Many people can't, and this is something to be aware of when you try. Don't push yourself too hard on this diet, or you will end up hurting yourself. If you pace yourself and eat well, you may be able to adjust and lose weight.

Some ideas for working out when you're doing the keto diet that are lower intensity are the following.

- Rowing

- Hiking

Gymnastics is also good for preventing injury and improving flexibility as well as improving how you move.

An example of a low-intensity workout that you can do is walking. This is easy to do, and it is great for losing weight. Swimming is another good activity though it straddles the fence. If you go lightly and keep it in the low-intensity area, then you are alright. If you push too hard it could be dangerous. When you are able to keep this thought in mind you will be able to perform exercises safely and make sure that they are working for you, not against you.

Chapter 2: Tips for Success

Routines are very important on this diet, and it's something that will help you stay healthy. As such, in this chapter, we are going to be giving you tips and tricks to make this diet work better for you and help you get an idea of routines that you can put in place for yourself.

Tip number one that is so important is DRINK WATER! This is absolutely vital for any diet that your on, and you need it if not on one as well. However, this vital tip is crucial on a keto diet because when you are eating fewer carbs, you are storing less water, meaning that you are going to get dehydrated very easily. You should aim for more than the daily amount of water however, remember that drinking too much water can be fatal as your kidneys can only handle so much as once. While this has mostly happened to soldiers in the military, it does happen to dieters as well, so it is something to be aware of.

Along with that same tip is to keep your electrolytes. You have three major electrolytes in your body. When you are on a keto diet, your body is reducing the amount of water that you store. It can be flushing out the electrolytes that your body needs as well, and this can make you sick. Some of the ways that you can fight this is by either salting your food or drinking bone broth. You can also eat pickled vegetables.

Eat when your hungry instead of snacking or eating constantly. This is also going to help, and when you focus on natural foods and health foods, this will help you even more. Eating processed foods is the worst thing you can do for fighting cravings, so you should really get into the routine of trying to eat whole foods instead.

Another routine that you can get into is setting a note somewhere that you can see it that will remind you of why you're doing this in the first place and why it's important to you. Dieting is hard, and you will have moments of weakness where you're wondering why you are doing this. Having a reminder will help you feel better, and it can really help with your perspective.

Tracking progress is something that straddles the fence. A Lot of people say that this helps a lot of people and you can celebrate your wins, however, as everyone is different and they have different goals, progress can be slower in some than others. This can cause others to be frustrated and sad, as well as wanting to give up. One of the most important things to remember is that while progress takes time, and you shouldn't get discouraged if you don't see results right away. With most diets, it takes at least a month to see any results. So don't get discouraged and keep trying if your body is saying that you can. If you can't, then you will need to talk to your doctor and see if something else is for you.

You should make it a daily routine to try and lower your stress. Stress will not allow you to get into ketosis, which is that state that keto wants to put you in. The reason for this being that stress increases the hormone known as cortisol in your blood, and it will prevent your body from being able to burn fats for energy. This is because your body has too much sugar in your blood. If you're going through a really high period of stress right now in your life, then this diet is not a great idea. Some great ideas for this would be getting into the habit or routine of taking the time to do something relaxing, such as walking and making sure that you're getting enough sleep, leads to the next routine that you need to do.

You need to get enough sleep. This is so important not just for your diet but also for your mind and body as well. Poor sleep also raises those stress hormones that can cause issues for you, so you need to get into the routine of getting seven hours of sleep at night on the minimum and nine hours if you can. If you're getting less than this, you need to change the routine you have in place right now and make sure that you establish a new routine where you are getting more sleep. As a result, your health and diet will be better.

Another routine that you need to get into is to give up diet soda and sugar substitutes. This is going to help you with your diet as well because diet soda can actually increase your sugar levels to a bad amount, and most diet sodas contain aspartame. This can be a carcinogen, so it's actually quite dangerous. Another downside is that using these sugar substitutes just makes you want more sugar later. Instead, you need to get into the habit of drinking water or sparkling water if you like the carbonation.

Staying consistent is another routine that you need to get yourself into. No matter what you are choosing to do, make sure it's something that you can actually do. Try a routine for a couple of weeks and make serious notes of mental and physical problems that you're going through as well as any emotional issues that come your way. Make changes as necessary until you find something that works well for you and that you can stick to. Remember that you need to give yourself time to get used to this and time to get used to changes before you give up on them.

Be honest with yourself, as well. This is another big tip for this diet. If you're not honest with yourself, this isn't going to work. Another reason that you need to be honest with yourself is if something isn't working you need to be able to understand that and change it. Are you giving yourself enough time to make changes? Are you pushing too hard? If so, you need to understand what is going on with yourself and how you need to deal with the changes that you're going through. Remember not to get upset or frustrated. This diet takes time, and you need to be able to be a little more patient to make this work effectively.

Getting into the routine of cooking for yourself is also going to help you so much on this diet. Eating out is fun, but honestly, on this diet, it can be hard to eat out. It is possible to do so with a little bit of special ordering and creativity, but you can avoid all the trouble by simply cooking for yourself. It saves time, and it saves a lot of cash.

This next topic falls into both the tip and routine category. Get into the habit of cleaning your kitchen. It's very hard to stick to a diet if your kitchen is dirty and full of junk food. Clear out the junk (donate it if you can, even though it's junk, there are tons of hungry people that would appreciate it) and replace all of the bad food with healthy keto food instead. Many people grab the carbs like crazy because they haven't cleared out their cabinets, and it's everywhere they look. Remember, with this diet, no soda, pasta, bread, candy, and things of that nature.

Replacing your food with healthy food and making a regular routine of cleaning your kitchen and keeping the bad food out is going to help you be more successful with your diet, which is what you want here.

Getting into the routine of having snacks on hand is a good idea as well. This keeps you from giving into temptation while your out, and you can avoid reaching for that junk food. You can make sure that they are healthy, and you will be sticking to your high-intensity diet, which is what you want. There are many different keto snacks that you can use for yourself and to eat. We will have a list of recipes in the following chapters to help this as well.

A good tip would be to use keto sticks or a glucose meter. This will give you feedback on whether your users do this diet right. The best option here is a glucose meter. It's expensive, but it's the most accurate. Be aware that if you use ketostix, they are cheaper, but the downside is that they are not accurate enough to help you. A perfect example is that they have a habit of telling people their ketone count is low when they are actually the opposite.

Try not to overeat as this will throw you out of where you need to be. Get into the routine of paying attention to what your eating and how much. If this is something that you're struggling with, try investing in a food scale. You will be able to see exactly what it is your eating and make sure that your understanding your portions and making sure you stay in ketosis.

Another tip is to make sure that you're improving your gut health. This is so important. Your gut is pretty much linked to every other system in your body, so make sure that this something that you want to take seriously. When you have healthy gut flora, your body's hormones, along with your insulin sensitivity and metabolic flexibility will all be more efficient. When your flexibility is functioning at an optimal level, your body is able to adapt to your diet easier. If it's not, then it will convert the fat your trying to use for energy into body fat.

Batch cooking or meal prepping is another routine that is a good thing to get into. This is an especially good routine for on the go women. When you cook in batches, you are able to make sure that you have meals that are ready to go, and you don't have to cook every single day, and you can save a lot of time as well. You will also be making your environment better for your diet because you're supporting your goals instead of working against them.

The last tip is to mention exercise again. Getting into the routine of exercising can boost your ketone levels, and it can help you with your issues on transitioning to keto. Exercises also use different types of energy for your fuel that you need. When your body gets rid of the glycogen storages, it needs other forms of energy, and it will turn into that energy that you need. Just remember to avoid exercises that are going to hurt you. Stay in the smaller exercises and lower intensity.

Following these tips and getting into these routines is going to help you stay on track and make sure that your diet will go as smoothly as it possibly can.

Part Two: 30 Day Meal Plan

Are you a busy mom that's on the go? Or maybe you work in an office, and you only get a small amount of time to eat? Whatever your situation is, we've got recipes that are easy to make and just as easy to take with you, so you don't have to worry about missing a meal or not having enough time to eat. Some of the recipes that we will be showing you in the following chapters can be done in as few as ten minutes! It doesn't get any easier than that.

We will show you breakfast recipes first and then go in order of the meals with snacks at the end. So let's get started! A side note for all of the recipes is that only you know what you need in terms of carbs, calories, fat, and so on. As such, you are free to mix and match based on your personal needs. As a special note, these recipes have nutritional information, and they are based on serving.

Chapter 3: Breakfast Recipes

Avocado and eggs

Time needed to prepare: 20 minutes

This will give you a single serving

What you need:

- 3 free-range eggs (use large)
- 3 thin slices of bacon (cut them into small pieces)
- A single tablespoon of butter (use salted)
- A single avocado (remove the stone and cut the avocado in half)

What you need to do:

1. Scoop out your flesh of avocado. Be sure to leave a half-inch around the avocado.
2. Put a saucepan on a heat that is low before adding in your butter.
3. While it's melting, crack your eggs and beat them.
4. Add your bacon to the pan and let them dry on their own for a few minutes before adding your eggs to the opposite side of your pan.
5. Stir frequently during your scrambling.
6. The bacon and eggs should both be finished five minutes after you have added the eggs to the pan.

7. If you have finished the eggs, first take them out before finishing the bacon.
8. Mix the bacon pieces and your eggs before adding them to the avocado halves.

Nutritional information:

- Calories-500
- Fiber-8 grams
- Protein-25 grams
- Carbs-11 grams
- Fat-40 grams

Lemon smoothie

You will need 5 minutes for this

You will get 4 servings for this

You will need:

- A third of a cup of lemon juice (freshly squeezed)
- A quarter of a cup of powdered Swerve Sweetener
- A third of a cup of water
- 2 cups of ice
- A cup of yogurt (Greek)
- A cup of raspberries (frozen)
- 2 ounces of cream cheese
- A single teaspoon zest from a lemon

What you need to do:

1. Get a blender.
2. Add all of your ingredients.
3. Blend until its a smooth consistency.

Nutritional information:

- Calories-148
- Fat-9.67 grams
- Fiber-1.06 grams
- Protein-5.41 grams
- Carbs-8.48 grams

Egg casserole

Time needed to prepare: 50 minutes

- The reason that this is on the list for women on the go is that you can make this the night before or early in the morning and it will give you eight servings which means that you can take servings with you and have leftovers and not have any cooking prep for other days.

This will give you eight servings

What you need:

- Half a dozen bacon slices (six)
- A dozen eggs (12 and use large)
- 10 ounces cheddar cheese (use shredded)
- 4 ounces of sour cream
- Cooking spray (use avocado oil spray)
- 4 ounces heavy whipping cream
- ⅓ of a cup of chopped green onions (this is optional but adds some great flavor to the dish)

What you need to do:

1. Preheat your oven to 350 degrees.
2. Cook your bacon on the stove before crumbling into bite-sized pieces after it has cooled, so you don't burn yourself.

3. Crack your eggs in a bowl before adding the cream.
4. Mix in a blender until it has combined well.
5. Spray a casserole pan with the spray before placing the cheese in a layer before adding the egg mix and bacon over the top.
6. Bake for thirty-five minutes.
7. Check it after a half-hour.
8. Remove from the oven when the edges have turned a color that looks golden brown.
9. Cool before cutting and placing your onions on top.

Nutritional Information:
- Calories-437
- Protein-43 grams
- Carbs-2 grams
- Fat-38 grams

As far as breakfast goes, this is a good one. You get a huge protein-packed breakfast, and it's got that fat you want as well. Just remember to be aware of your numbers. If you eat this much protein, now be careful to make sure that you're not going over later.

Broccoli Bread

This will take 35 minutes in total to prepare

It will give you ten servings

What you will need:

- A single cup of cheddar cheese (make sure that it is shredded)
- 5 eggs (make sure that they are beaten)
- 3 ½ tablespoons of flour (you should use coconut)
- 2 tsp of baking powder
- ¾ of a cup of broccoli florets (you need to make sure that they are raw, fresh, and chopped)

What you need to do:

1. Heat your oven to 350.
2. Spray a pan with cooking spray.
3. Mix all of your ingredients in a bowl before pouring it in the pan.
4. Bake for half an hour.
5. Add five minutes if necessary. It should be golden and puffed.
6. Slice into servings.

If you want to reheat this, all you have to do is use the microwave.

Nutritional information:

- Calories-90
- Fat-6 grams
- Protein- 6 grams
- Carbs- 2 grams
- Fiber-1 gram

Pizza

Time you will need: 25 minutes

You will be able to get two servings from this

What you will need:

- 4 eggs
- 2 cups of cauliflower (make sure that it is grated)
- 2 tablespoons of flour (make sure it's coconut)
- A single tablespoon of husk powder (use psyllium and make sure it's a brand that is mold-free)
- Olive oil, avocado, spinach, spices and herbs, and salmon (smoked) for toppings for the pizza to offer flavor and nutrients

What you need to do:

1. Heat your oven to 350 before lining a pizza tray with parchment.
2. Add all of the ingredients except what you will be using for the top of the pizza and mix into a bowl.
3. Set it aside.
4. Let it sit for at least five minutes, so the husk and flour are able to absorb the liquid that they need to.

5. Pour the base of the pizza in the pan. Go slow and be careful before molding it into a round pizza crust and make sure that it is even.
6. Let it bake for a quarter of an hour (fifteen minutes).
7. It should be fully cooked and golden brown.
8. Remove and top with your chosen items.

Nutritional information:

- Calories -454
- Fat-31 grams
- Carbs- 26 grams
- Protein-22 grams
- Fiber-17.2 grams

Pizza for breakfast? Yes, please! Now you will see that the carbs for this breakfast is a little high. This is why you can play with what you put on the pizza to create less carbs if you like.

Donuts

Time you will need for this: 40 minutes

You will be able to get 6 servings with this

What you will need:

- 2 eggs (make sure they are large)
- A single cup of flour (almond and blanched)
- A single tablespoon of cinnamon
- ½ of a teaspoon of vanilla extract
- 2 teaspoons of baking powder (use gluten-free)
- ⅓ of a cup of erythritol
- ¼ of a cup of butter (this will need to be solid when you measure, then melted and it needs to be unsalted as well)
- ¼ of a cup of milk (it needs to be almond and unsweetened)

For the coating for the donuts:

- 3 tablespoons of butter (same steps as above. Measure it solid, melt it and then make sure that you have chosen a butter that is unsalted)
- 1 teaspoon of cinnamon
- ½ of a cup of erythritol

What you need to do:

1. Heat your oven to 350 before greasing a donut pan and greasing it well.
2. Mix your ingredients (the dry ones) in a bowl.
3. In a separate bowl, mix in your eggs, milk, butter, and vanilla extract.
4. Mix the wet bowl into the dry bowl.
5. When you have made the batter, transfer it into the donut spots in the donut pan. Don't fill them all the way. Fill it a little more than half.
6. Bake for 25 minutes. If you have a silicone pan, you will have to go longer.
7. When it is done, they should be a nice and even golden brown color.
8. Let cool.
9. Remove from pan.
10. In a bowl, mix the dry ingredients for the topping.
11. When the donuts are cool, remove them from the mold and brush the side of the donut with the butter before pressing the mix of dry ingredients on top. It should create a crust.
12. Repeat for the other five donuts before eating.

Nutritional information:

- Calories-257
- Fat-25 grams
- Protein-6 grams
- Fiber-2 grams
- Carbs-5 grams

Crepes

You will need 15 minutes for this

You will be able to get 2 from this

What you will need:

- A single tablespoon husk powder (use a psyllium version)
- A single tablespoon of sweetener (if you are sticking to the tip that we have told you above you can cut this part out)
- ⅓ of a cup of water (make sure it's boiling)
- 3 eggs
- 3 tablespoons of flour (use coconut)

For the filling of the crepes:

- ½ of a cup of berries (raspberries or strawberries)
- A single ounce of dark chocolate (use the tip we gave you in the previous chapters)
- ½ of a tablespoon of oil or butter (if you are using oil use coconut)

What you need to do:

1. Mix the flour, husk, sweetener if you are going to use it, and the eggs into a boil.
2. Mix in your water and make sure it combines well.

3. In a pan that is nonstick, add in a single tablespoon of oil and turn up the heat to a medium level.
4. Add in no more than half of the liquid for the crepes and allow them to cook until the edges have turned brown.
5. Flip it over.
6. Cook until golden brown.
7. This should take no more than five minutes per crepe.
8. Repeat until all the dough is finished.
9. If you have chosen to add berries and chocolate, then you will need to melt your chocolate first before adding a spoonful to the middle of the crepe and adding the berries.
10. Close it up.
11. If you choose top with additional chocolate or berries for extra flavor.

Nutritional information:

- Calories-167
- Carbs-5 grams
- Protein-7 grams
- Fat-12 grams
- Fiber-5 grams

Omelette

You will need 17 minutes for this

You will get 2 servings for this

What you need:

- 7 ounces of spinach (frozen)
- Half of a dozen large eggs (six)
- 2 tablespoons of milk (you should use heavy cream or almond milk)
- 2 teaspoons of oil for frying (we are going to use olive oil)
- A single tablespoon of herbs (chives or parsley is good, but you need to make sure that they are fresh)
- A quarter of a cup of grated sharp cheddar
- A quarter of a cup of grated parmesan cheese
- A quarter of a cup of crumbled, mild feta cheese
- A single handful of kale that is chopped (discard the stems)
- A half of a cup of ricotta cheese
- Pepper for taste

What you will need to do:

1. Make sure that there is no liquid in your spinach. If there is, then you will need to squeeze it out. You should have a small handful left.

2. Chop the spinach finely then do the same with the kale (a food processor makes this easier and quicker).
3. Add the parmesan cheese along with cheddar, eggs, and milk and mix it well so it will combine well.
4. Mix the herbs, feta, and ricotta in a separate bowl and then season with pepper.
5. Place the bowl to the side.
6. Heat a single teaspoon of olive oil in a pan that is non-stick.
7. Pour in half of the egg mix you made.
8. On medium-high heat fry until just set.
9. Add half of the ricotta mix on top before folding the omelette over.
10. Be careful when you do this.
11. Place a lid over the pan and then cook for another minute so that your filling is warmed.
12. Repeat for the second omelette.

Nutritional information:

- Calories-522
- Fat-34.7 grams
- Fiber-2.4 grams
- Protein-44 grams
- Carbs-10.3 grams

Cheesy Bread

You will need 30 minutes for this

You will get 8 servings from this

You will need:

- A single egg
- A single tablespoon of cream cheese
- ¾ of a cup of mozzarella cheese
- A single teaspoon of basil
- A single tablespoon of garlic powder.
- 2 tablespoons of flour (you should use almond)

You will need to do the following:

1. Heat your oven to 350
2. Melt your cream cheese and cheese
3. Mix in the flour and your egg.
4. Get a baking sheet and line it with parchment paper.
5. Flatten your mixture on top of the sheet.
6. Sprinkle your garlic on the mixture.
7. Bake for twenty minutes.

Nutritional information:

Serving size is one.

- Calories-56
- Protein-3.6 grams
- Fat-4.5 grams
- Fiber-0.2 grams
- Carbs-0.8 grams

Strawberries to the rescue!

You will need 5 minutes for this

You will get one serving from this

You will need:

- 2/3 of a cup of water
- Half a cup of strawberries (you can use either use frozen or fresh)
- Half a teaspoon of vanilla extract
- A third of a cup of coconut milk that is unsweetened.

What you need to do:

1. Place all of the ingredients in your blender.
2. Blend it all until smooth.
3. Pour in a glass.

Nutritional information:

- Calories-149
- Carbs-8 grams
- Protein-6 grams
- Fiber-2 grams
- Fat-11 grams

Chia smoothie

You will need 5 minutes for this

You will get 4 serving from this

You will need:

- A single cup of blueberries (frozen)
- A half-cup of coconut cream
- A single cup of yogurt (use Greek and full fat)
- 2 tablespoons of coconut oil
- A single cup of almond milk that is unsweetened
- 2 tablespoons of sweetener (we're going with Swerve)
- 2 tablespoons of chia seeds (ground)

What you need to do:

1. Using a blender add all of your ingredients before blending until it is smooth.
2. Pour into glasses.

Nutritional information:

- Calories-249
- Fat-21.07 grams
- Fiber-3.55 grams
- Carbs-7.71 grams
- Protein-6.23 grams

Protein smoothie

You will need 5 minutes for this

You will get one serving from this

You will need:

- A single cup of ice
- Half of an avocado
- A single cup of spinach that's fresh
- 10 drops or 12 drops of Stevia Peppermint Sweet Drops (sweet leaf liquid drops)
- A single scoop of whey protein powder
- A half-cup of almond milk that is unsweetened
- A quarter teaspoon of peppermint extract

What you need to do:

1. Place everything but the drops, extract, and ice in the blender and blend.
2. Add the extract, ice, and drops.
3. Blend until its thick.

Nutritional information:

- Calories-293
- Fat-15 grams
- Carbs-11 grams
- Fiber- 7 grams
- Protein-28 grams

Blueberry smoothie

You will need 11 minutes for this

You will get one serving from this

You will need:

- A single cup of coconut milk
- A single teaspoon of vanilla extract
- A single teaspoon of coconut oil
- A quarter cup of blueberries

What you need to do:

1. Using a blender, blend until everything is smooth.

Nutritional information:

- Calories-215
- Fat-10 grams
- Carbs-7 grams
- Protein-23 grams
- Fiber-3 grams

Spinach smoothie

You will need 5 minutes for this

You will get one serving from this

You will need:

- 4 ice cubes
- A single tablespoon of mint (fresh)
- Half of a cup of cucumber (you will need to peel it before seeding it)
- A single cup of water (make sure it is filtered)
- A single cup of spinach (fresh)
- 4 ounces of coconut milk (canned and full fat)
- A single scoop of whey protein (grass-fed and naturally nourished)

What you need to do:

1. Get a blender.
2. Blend.
3. When smooth, pour in a glass.

Nutritional information:

- Calories-360
- Fat-24 grams
- Protein-27 grams
- Carbs-10 grams

Almond smoothie

You will need 5 minutes for this

You will get one serving from this

You will need:

- A single tablespoon of almond butter
- A single pinch of cinnamon
- A single teaspoon of vanilla extract
- A few ice cubes
- A single cup of almond milk (unsweetened)
- A single scoop of whey protein (use grass-fed and make sure that it is naturally nourished)

What you need to do:

1. Combine everything in a blender but the whey protein.
2. Once it's nice and mixed whip in your protein only for a moment to incorporate.

Nutritional information:

- Calories-255
- Fat-14 grams
- Carbs-7 grams
- Protein- 29 grams

Avocado smoothie

You will need 2 minutes for this

You will get 2 servings from this

What you need:

- A single avocado (make sure it is ripe. You will peel and remove the pit)
- A cup and a third of water
- 2 tablespoons of sugar substitute (make sure its low carb)
- 2 to 3 tablespoons of juice from a lemon
- Half of a cup of raspberries (unsweetened and frozen)

What you need to do:

1. Place all of your ingredients in a blender.
2. Blend your ingredients until they are smooth.
3. Pour into a glass.

Nutritional value:

- Calories-227
- Fat-20 grams
- Fiber-8.8 grams
- Carbs-12.8 grams

Protein-2.5 grams

Pumpkin smoothie

You will need 5 minutes for this

You will get one serving with this

You will need:

- 3 tablespoons of puree (use pumpkin)
- A single teaspoon of tea (use loose chai)
- A single teaspoon of vanilla (alcohol-free)
- 3/4 of a cup of coconut milk (full fat)
- Half of a cup of avocado (use frozen)
- Half a teaspoon of pumpkin pie spice
- Half of an avocado (fresh. If fresh isn't available you can use frozen)

What you need to do:

1. Get a blender.
2. Add everything but avocado to the blender.
3. Blend until everything is smooth.
4. Add your avocado and blend.
5. Keep blending until broken apart.
6. Serve with the spice on top.

Nutritional information:

- Calories-726
- Fat-69.8 gram
- Fiber-8.2 grams
- Carbs-19.5 grams
- Protein-5.5 grams

Tumeric time!

You will need 5 minutes for this

You will get one serving for this

You will need:

- A single tablespoon of turmeric (use ground)
- 6.7 ounces of coconut milk (use full fat)
- A single teaspoon of cinnamon (use ground)
- 6.7 ounces of almond milk (unsweetened)
- A single teaspoon of granulated sweetener.
- A single tablespoon of chia seeds for the top of the smoothie
- A single tablespoon of coconut oil
- A single teaspoon of ginger (ground)

What you need to do:

1. Get a blender.
2. Place all of the ingredients in the blender, except chia seeds.
3. Add some ice if needed.
4. Blend until everything is smooth.
5. Sprinkle chia seeds to the top.

Nutritional information:

- Calories- 600
- Fat-56 grams
- Carbs-6 grams
- Protein-7 grams

Sausage sandwich

You will need 10 minutes for this

You will get one serving from this

What you need:

- A single tablespoon of cream cheese
- 2 sausage patties
- A single egg
- 2 tablespoons of cheddar (sharp)
- A quarter of a medium avocado (sliced)
- A quarter of a teaspoon to a half of a teaspoon of sriracha.

What you need to do:

1. Get a skillet.
2. Turn your heat to medium.
3. Cook sausages as the packet says to.
4. Set aside.
5. Mix your cheese with your sriracha.
6. Set it to the side.
7. Cook your egg into a small omelet.
8. Fill the omelet with cheese mix and assemble your sandwich

Nutritional information:

- Calories- 603
- Fat- 54 grams
- Protein-22 grams
- Carbs-7 grams

A taste of Italy omelet style

You will need 10 minutes for this

You will get 2 servings from this

What you need:

- Half a dozen eggs (six)
- 2 tablespoons of olive oil
- A single tablespoon of basil (fresh and chopped)
- 5 ounces of mozzarella cheese (fresh and diced)
- 3 tomatoes (cherry. Cut them in half)

What you need to do:

1. Get a bowl.
2. Crack your eggs into the bowl.
3. Add salt and pepper for taste.
4. Whisk with a fork and do it well. This lets the ingredients combine.
5. Add in your basil.
6. Stir.
7. Get a large frying pan.
8. Heat oil in the pan.
9. Fry your tomatoes for a few minutes.
10. Pour the egg mixture on the tomatoes.
11. After the batter has become slightly firm, add your cheese.

12. Turn down your heat and let your omelet set.
13. It is now ready to eat.

Nutritional information:

- Calories-534
- Fat-43 grams
- Fiber-1 gram
- Carbs-4 grams
- Protein-33 grams

Pancakes

You will need 12 minutes for this

You will get 4 servings from this

What you need:

- 2 ounces of cream cheese
- 2 eggs
- A single teaspoon of granulated sugar substitute
- Half of a teaspoon of cinnamon

What you need to do:

1. Put all of your ingredients in a blender.
2. Blend until its smooth.
3. Let it sit for 2 minutes.
4. Pour a quarter of the mix into a pan that is hot. The pan needs to be greased with butter.
5. Cook for 2 minutes .
6. It should be golden.
7. Flip it.
8. Cook another minute.
9. Repeat until the mix is gone.

Nutritional information:

- Calories-344
- Fat-29 grams
- Carbs-3 carbs
- Protein-17 carbs

Muffins

You will need only one minute for this

You will get one serving for this

You will need:

- A single egg
- A pinch of baking soda
- A pinch of salt
- 2 tablespoons of flour (coconut)

What you need to do:

1. Get a large coffee mug.
2. Grease it with oil (coconut) or butter if you don't have oil.
3. Mix everything together.
4. Make sure you have no lumps.
5. Cook in the microwave on high.
6. Do this for 45 seconds to a single minute.
7. Cut in two pieces, and you have a muffin.

Nutritional information:

- Calories-113
- Fat-6 grams
- Fiber-3 grams
- Protein-7 grams
- Carbs- 5 grams

Hearty breakfast

You will need 15 minutes for this

You will get one serving for this

You will need:

- 2 eggs (organic, pastured, large)
- 4 bacon strips (pastured, and uncured)
- A single avocado (large. You need to peel it before cutting it in slices)
- A quarter teaspoon of sea salt

What you need to do:

1. Put the bacon and avocado in a non-toxic ceramic frying pan on medium heat.
2. Cook three minutes before flipping both.
3. Remove both from the pan and place to the side.
4. Make sure that they are keeping warm.
5. Leave the drippings in the pan.
6. Crack your eggs into the pan.
7. You will be frying them for two to three minutes.
8. Flip your egg and fry until it is how you like.

Nutritional information:

- Calories-313
- Fat-26 grams
- Fiber- 6 grams
- Carbs-2.6 grams
- Protein-13 grams

Avocado lemon smoothie

You will need minutes for this

You will get servings from this

What you need:

- A simple cup of water that is cold
- Half of a cup of cilantro
- A single cup of spinach (use baby spinach)
- A single cup of avocado (use frozen)
- Peeled ginger (use a one-inch ginger)
- Half of a peeled lemon to one whole peeled lemon
- 3/4 of an English cucumber (it needs to be peeled)

What you need to do:

1. Get a blender that is high speed.
2. Add everything in the blender.
3. Blend until everything is smooth.
4. You need to store it in an airtight container.
5. It will last no longer than three days.

Nutritional information:

- Calories-148
- Fat-11 grams
- Fiber-6 grams
- Carbs- 13 grams
- Protein-2 grams

Cucumber smoothie

You will need 5 minutes for this

You will get 2 servings from this

What you need:

- 8 ounces of water
- A single cup of sliced cucumber
- 2 ounces of avocado (make sure it is ripe)
- A half teaspoon of liquid stevia (lemon)
- A single teaspoon of lemon juice
- 2 teaspoons of Green Tea powder (use match)
- Half a cup of ice
- A single teaspoon of juice from a lemon

What you need to do:

1. Pour your powder and water into a blender.
2. Blend to let the two combine.
3. Add the rest of your ingredients and blend. You should blend on high until it has become smooth.

Nutritional information:

- Calories-69
- Fat-4.6 grams
- Fiber- 3.4 grams
- Protein-2 grams
- Carbs-6.8 grams

Dragon fruit smoothie

You will need 5 minutes for this

You will get one serving from this

You will need:

- Half of a dragon fruit (small)
- Half of a cup of coconut milk
- A single galia melon wedge (small wedge)
- A single tablespoon of chia seeds
- 3 drops to 6 drops liquid stevia extract
- A single scoop of whey protein powder (vanilla)
- Try to find organic if you can for these ingredients

What you need to do:

1. Measure your ingredients and place them in a blender.
2. Pulse in your blender until smooth and ready to drink.

Nutritional information:

- Calories-403
- Fat-28.6 grams
- Protein-24.6
- Carbs-17 grams
- Fiber-4.9 grams

Egg smoothie

You will need 5 minutes for this

You will get one serving from this

You will need:

- A quarter cup of whipping cream (heavy)
- A half teaspoon of cinnamon
- A single egg (large one)
- 4 Cloves (ground)
- A single teaspoon of Erythritol

What you need to do:

1. Put all of your ingredients into a blender.
2. Blend.
3. If you do this for 60 seconds, you will get a bit of froth at the top.

Nutritional information:

- Calories-320
- Fat-30 grams
- Carbs-8 grams
- Fiber- 2 grams
- Protein-6 grams

Burrito

You will need 7minutes for this

You will get 1 serving from this (one burrito)

What you need:

- 2 eggs (use medium)
- A single tablespoon of butter
- 2 tablespoons of full fat cream

What you need to do:

1. Get a bowl.
2. Whisk the eggs in the bowl along with the cream.
3. Get a frying pan.
4. Melt your butter in the pan.
5. Pour in egg mix.
6. Swirl your frying pan until your burrito mixture is both thin and spread evenly.
7. Place a lid over the burrito pan.
8. Cook two minutes.
9. Lift burrito from pan.
10. Put on a plate.
11. If you choose to fill with veggies!

Nutritional information:

- Calories-331
- Fat-30 grams
- Carbs-1 gram
- Protein-11 grams

Let's get back to basics

You will need 10 minutes for this

You will get 2 servings from this

What you need:

- Half a dozen eggs (six)
- 3 ounces of butter
- 7 ounces of cheddar cheese (use shredded)

What you need to do:

1. Whisk your eggs. When they are frothy (slightly) and smooth, you can continue.
2. Blend in 3.5 ounces of cheddar (half)
3. Get a frying pan.
4. Melt your butter.
5. The pan needs to be hot for you to do this.
6. Pour in your egg mix.
7. Let it sit for a few moments.
8. Lower your heat.
9. Continue to cook until the egg mix has almost cooked through.
10. Add the rest of the cheese.
11. Fold omelet.
12. Place on a plate after removing from the stove.

Nutritional information:

- Calories-897
- Fat-80 grams
- Carbs-4 grams
- Protein-40 grams

Mocha smoothie

You will need 5minutes for this

You will get 3 servings from this

What you need:

- A single teaspoon of vanilla extract
- Half of a cup of coconut milk.
- A cup and a half of almond milk that is unsweetened
- 2 teaspoons of regular instant coffee crystals
- 3 tablespoons of a granulated stevia/erythritol blend
- 3 tablespoons of cocoa powder that is unsweetened
- A single avocado cut in half (the pit needs to be removed)

What you need to do:

1. Place everything in a blender except the avocado.
2. Blend it until it becomes smooth.
3. Add in your avocado by scooping it in.
4. Blend until smooth again.
5. Pour into 3 glasses.

Nutritional information:

- Calories-176
- Fat-16
- Carbs-10
- Fiber-6 grams
- Protein-3 grams

Chapter 4: Lunch Recipes

Lemon soup

You will need 15 minutes for this

You will get roughly 6 servings from this (possibly less)

What you need:

- 4 cups of water
- 2 tablespoons of lemon juice
- 2 cups of almond milk (unsweetened)
- ¾ of a cup of parmesan cheese
- 2.5 to 3 pounds of broccoli florets

What you need to do:

1. Get a large saucepan and then place your water and broccoli inside.
2. Cover the pan and cook on medium-high heat.
3. Do this until your broccoli is tender.
4. Reserve on the cups of the cooking liquid, but you can throw the rest away.
5. Add in half of the broccoli to a blender.
6. Add in the liquid you saved and the milk as well.
7. Blend until it's nice and smooth.
8. Return the mix to your pot and then add the parmesan along with your juice.
9. Heat it until it is hot.

Nutritional information:

- Calories-85
- Fat-3.1 grams
- Carbs-10.3 grams
- Protein-6.8 grams
- Fiber-4.0 grams

Caper salad

You will need 5 minutes for this

You will get 4 servings from this

You will need:

- Four ounces tuna (make sure that it is in olive oil)
- A single tablespoon of capers
- 2 tablespoons of creme fraiche
- Half a cup of mayo
- Half of a finely chopped leek
- Half a teaspoon of chili flakes

What you need to do:

1. Drain tuna.
2. Mix everything together.
3. Season

Nutritional information:

- Calories-271
- Fat-26 grams
- Carbs- 1 grams
- Protein 8 grams

Salmon with cucumber

You will need 20 minutes for this

You will get 4 servings from this

What you need for the Salmon:

- A single pound and a half of salmon (and it needs to be in pieces)
- 2 tablespoons of oil (use olive)
- 2 tablespoons of seasoning (use tendori)

What you need for the sauce:

- 3/4 of a cup of mayo
- 2 cloves of minced garlic
- Juice from half a lime
- Half of a cucumber (make sure that it is shredded)

What you need for your salad:

- 5 ounces of lettuce (use romaine)
- 3 scallions
- The juice from a lime
- A single bell pepper (use yellow)
- 2 avocados

What you need to do:

1. Heat your oven to 350.
2. Mix the seasoning with oil.
3. Cover your salmon with the mixture.
4. Bake for fifteen minutes minimum and twenty minutes maximum.
5. Your salmon should flake easily with a fork.
6. Mix everything together but the scallions, peppers, avocados, and lime juice. With the shredded cucumber, the water needs to be squeezed out.
7. Chop the remaining ingredients.
8. Place on your plate.
9. Over the top, drizzle your juice from the lime.
10. Next to them, place your salad and put the salmon on top.
11. Then top it with it the sauce.

Nutritional information:

- Calories-886
- Fat-76 grams
- Protein-38 grams
- Carbs-8 grams
- Fiber-9 grams

Pumpkin soup

You will need 20 minutes for this

You will get 6 servings for this

You will need:

- 15 ounces of puree (pumpkin)
- Half a teaspoon of pepper
- Half a teaspoon of salt
- 4 cups of broth (go with chicken)
- A single teaspoon of thyme (make sure it's fresh)
- Half a teaspoon of garlic powder
- Half a cup of heavy cream

What you need to do:

1. In a saucepan, combine everything but the heavy cream.
2. Stir, so they combine properly.
3. Bring to a boil.
4. Reduce heat and let it simmer for ten minutes.
5. Remove from heat before adding the cream.

Nutritional information:

- Calories-120
- Fat-9 grams
- Fiber-2 grams
- Carbs-7 grams
- Protein-2 grams

Let's grill some shrimp

You will need 40 minutes for this

You will get 4 servings for this

You will need:

- A single garlic clove that is small
- A single tablespoon of toasted pine nuts
- 2 tablespoons of oil (we're going with olive)
- A single tablespoon of lemon juice from a lemon
- Half of a cup of packed basil
- A single pound of peeled and deveined shrimp
- 2 tablespoons grated parmesan

What you need to do:

1. Get a blender.
2. Pulse all of your ingredients except the shrimp in blender.
3. Let the shrimp marinate in the mix.
4. Do this for 20 minutes. If you have time, do it overnight in your refrigerator.
5. Skewer your shrimp and grill.
6. You will do this over a medium-high heat until cooked thoroughly.
7. This should take 3 minutes for each side.

Nutritional information:

- Calories-184
- Fat-11 grams
- Carbs-2 grams
- Protein-18 grams

Egg roll with a twist

You will need 30 minutes for this

You will get 4 servings from this

You will need:

- A single pound of ground pork
- A single white diced onion
- A single teaspoon of ginger (grated)
- 2 minced garlic cloves
- 12 ounces of a coleslaw mix
- 2 teaspoons of apple cider vinegar
- 2 tablespoons of chopped green onion
- 2 tablespoons of sesame oil
- 3 tablespoons coconut aminos

What you need to do:

1. Get a large skillet.
2. Turn heat to medium.
3. Bown your pork
4. When it is cooked, you can set it to the side.
5. Be sure to discard all of the fat.
6. With the skillet, you just used heat your oil on medium heat.
7. Using the same skillet, heat the oil on medium heat.
8. Put the garlic, ginger, and onion in the skillet.
9. Do this until the onion is translucent and is fragrant.

10. Pour your coleslaw mix in along with the aminos and vinegar.
11. Stir well so it can combine.
12. Saute for five minutes. The cabbage should have reduced in size. Your carrots should also be softened.
13. Reincorporate your pork and stir so it can combine.
14. Saute for another minute.
15. Remove from heat.
16. Top with your onions.

Nutritional information:

- Calories-351
- Fat-15.8 grams
- Carbs-15.8 grams
- Fiber-2.6 grams
- Protein-38.2 grams

Baked fish with sauce

You will need 20 minutes for this

You will get 2 servings from this

What you need:

- A teaspoon of garlic paste
- Whitefish fillets (use 150 gram fish. You need 2 of them)
- A single tablespoon of oil (use olive)
- A single broccolini bunch
- A single lemon
- 100 grams of butter

What you need to do:

1. Preheat your oven to 428F.
2. Get a baking dish.
3. Line it with baking paper.
4. Finely grate the rind of the lemon.
5. Cut half of the lemon. They need to be in small segments.
6. Pat your fish dry.
7. Drizzle the fish with half of the rind and olive oil.
8. Bake for a minimum of twelve minutes and a maximum of fourteen. It should be cooked through. It should also be able to just fall apart.

9. Steam broccolini until its just tender. This should be done in a microwave for four minutes.
10. Drain it.
11. Place it to the side so it can dry.
12. Get a frying pan.
13. Turn the heat to medium.
14. Heat your butter for four minutes. It should be golden or almost golden.
15. Add the rest of the rind and your garlic.
16. Cook for another sixty seconds.
17. Stir in your segments of lemon and the broccolini.
18. Top the fish with your sauce and broccolini.

Nutritional information:

- Calories-476
- Fat-47 grams
- Fiber-2 grams
- Carbs-12 grams
- Protein- 19 grams

Subs

You will need 10 minutes for this

You will get 8 servings from this

What you need:

- 4 green onions (be sure to slice in half)
- 2 avocados (remove the pit, peel it and slice it)
- 2 leaves of lettuce (use iceberg)
- 9 ounces of ham (use Italian style)
- 5 and a half ounces of genoa salami
- 5 and a half of salami (use soppressata)
- 4 and a half ounces of prosciutto

What you need to do:

1. Place a slice a ham slice on a cutting board
2. Add a piece of prosciutto.
3. Add four pieces of salami.
4. Make a square shape with your layers.
5. Add some avocado (just a couple of slices)
6. Add a green onion piece.
7. Add a piece of lettuce to the far side of your meat stack that you have made.
8. Roll the ingredients into a roll.

Nutritional information:

- Calories-270
- Fiber-22 grams
- Fat-3.8 grams
- Carbs-6.3 grams
- Protein-18.6 grams

Tuna salad

You will need 10 minutes for this

You will get one serving from this

You will need:

- One sliced green onion
- 2 cups of greens (mixed)
- Half of a diced avocado
- A single diced tomato (use a large one)
- A quarter cup of chopped fresh mint
- A quarter cup fresh chopped parsley
- 10 large pitted kalamata olives
- A single can of chunk light tuna (make sure it is in water and drain it)
- A single small sliced zucchini (slice it lengthwise)
- A single tablespoon of balsamic vinegar
- A single tablespoon of extra virgin olive oil

What you need to do:

1. Get a skillet (cast iron).
2. Grill your zucchini slices. Do it on both sides in a sizzling hot skillet.
3. Remove from your pan.
4. Let it cool for a few moments.
5. Cut into pieces.
6. Get a bowl.
7. Put all of the ingredients in a bowl.

8. Stir it together.

Nutritional information:

- Calories-563
- Fat-30.9 grams
- Carbs-37.5 grams
- Protein- 41.8 grams
- Fiber-15 grams

Taco time

You will need 45 minutes for this

You will get 8 servings from this

You will need:

- A single pound of ground beef
- Half a dozen eggs (six and use large ones)
- A single cup of heavy cream
- 2 minced garlic cloves
- 3 tablespoons of taco seasoning
- A single cup cheese (shredded and cheddar)

What you need to do:

1. Preheat your oven to 350.
2. Get a pie pan that is 9 inches.
3. Grease the pan.
4. Get a skillet that is large.
5. Turn your heat to medium.
6. Brown ground beef until there is no pink left.
7. This should take approximately seven minutes. Make sure there are no clumps.
8. Add the seasoning and stir until it has been combined.
9. Reduce your heat to medium-low. Cook for another few minutes longer.
10. Your sauce should be thickened.

11. Place your beef in the pan before spreading it out.
12. Get a bowl.
13. Combine the garlic, cream, and eggs.
14. If you like salt and pepper, add a sprinkle.
15. Pour the mix over your beef.
16. Sprinkle the cheese over the top.
17. Bake for a half-hour.
18. The center needs to be set, and your cheese should be browned.
19. Remove from oven.
20. Let your dish sit for five minutes.
21. Slice and you are ready to eat.

Nutritional information:

- Calories-370
- Fat-27.8 grams
- Carbs-2.14 grams
- Protein-24.1 grams

Cabbage plate

You will need 10 minutes for this

You will get 2 servings for this

What you need:

- 10 ounces of bacon
- 2 ounces of butter
- A single pound of green cabbage

You will need to do the following:

- Chop your ingredients into small pieces (not butter)
- Get a skillet.
- Fry your bacon over medium heat until it is crisp.
- Add the cabbage and butter .
- Fry it until it has become golden and soft.

Nutritional information:

- Calories-850
- Carbs-9 grams
- Fiber-6 grams
- Fat- 79 grams
- Protein-21 grams

Let's get those veggies!

You will need a half an hour for this

You will get 2 servings from this

What you need:

- A third of an eggplant
- Half a lemon(you want the juice)
- 10 olives (black)
- Half of a zucchini
- 5 ounces of cheese (use cheddar) a quarter of a cup of olive oil
- Half a cup of mayo
- A single ounce of a leafy green
- 2 tablespoons of almonds

What you need to do:

1. Slice your eggplant into slices a half-inch thick.
2. Do the same with your zucchini. The slices should also be lengthwise.
3. Sprinkle salt on both sides of the vegetables you have cut and then let them sit for a maximum of ten minutes and a minimum of 5.
4. Preheat your oven to 450 degrees.
5. Use paper towels to pat your vegetables until dry on the surface.
6. Get a baking sheet.
7. Line it with parchment paper.

8. Brush olive oil over the top before sprinkling pepper over them to add flavor.
9. Bake for fifteen minutes minimum and twenty at the maximum.
10. They should appear golden Bryan on both sides. Remember to flip halfway through.
11. Place on a plate and pour the juice and oil over the top.
12. Serve with the rest of your vegetables and arrange them how you like them.

Nutritional information:

- Calories-1013
- Fat-99 grams
- Fiber-6 grams
- Carbs-9 grams
- Protein-21 grams

Chicken plate

You will need 5 minutes for this

You will get two servings from this

You will need:

- A single pound of rotisserie chicken
- 2 ounces of lettuce
- 7 ounces of cheese (use feta)
- 2 tomatoes
- 10 olives (black)
- A third of a cup of olive oil

What you need to do:

1. Slice your veggies and put them on a plate
2. Add the other ingredients together on the plate.
3. Place the oil in a small dish in the middle, or pour over the top.
4. You can sprinkle pepper and salt over the top if you like.

Nutritional information:

- Calories-1194
- Fiber-2 grams
- Fat-102 grams
- Carbs-3 grams
- Protein-62 grams

Mushroom plate

You will need 15 minutes for this

You will get 2 servings from this

You will need:

- 10 olives (use green)
- 10 ounces of cheese (you need to use halloumi)
- 10 ounces of mushrooms
- 3 ounces of butter

What you need to do:

1. Your mushrooms need to be clean.
2. Rinse them and make sure that they are before trimming them.
3. Cut them into pieces.
4. Heat up a dollop of butter in a pan for frying.
5. Turn the heat to medium.
6. Fry your mushrooms for no longer than five minutes and no less than three minutes. They should be a golden brown color.
7. While your frying your mushrooms, fry your cheese on the other side of the pan.
8. You can fry the cheese on both sides for a couple of minutes.
9. Stir the mushrooms occasionally while they are frying.
10. The heat should be lowered toward the end.

11. When your ready to eat, place the olives around the cheese.

Nutritional information:

- Calories-830
- Fat-74 grams
- Fiber-2 grams
- Carbs-7 grams
- Protein-36 grams

Italian time

You will need 5 minutes for this

You will get two servings from this

You will need:

- 7 ounces of mozzarella cheese (make sure it's fresh)
- 10 olives (green)
- A third of a cup of olive oil
- 2 tomatoes
- 7 ounces of sliced prosciutto

What you need to do:

1. Arrange all of the items on your plate in any fashion you like.
2. Place the oil in a small dish and place it in the center.

Nutritional information:

- Calories-822
- Fiber-3 grams
- Carbs-4 grams
- Protein-40 grams
- Fat-69 grams

Eggplant plate

You will need 10 minutes for this

You will get 2 servings from this

What you need:

- A single eggplant
- 10 ounces cheese (use halloumi)
- 3 ounces of butter
- 10 olives (black)

What you need to do:

1. Cut your eggplant in half (lengthwise).
2. Cut into slices. (Go for a half-inch in thickness).
3. Heat butter in a pan for frying.
4. Place eggplant alone on one side and the cheese on the other.
5. On a medium-high heat fry for seven minutes maximum and five minimum.
6. Remember to flip the cheese after three minutes. It should be golden brown on both sides.
7. Stir the vegetables once every few minutes.
8. When you are ready to eat, place your olives around the dish.

Nutritional information:

- Calories-829
- Fiber-8 grams
- Fat-72 grams
- Carbs-11 grams
- Protein-32 grams

Avocado, anyone?

You will need 10 minutes for this

You will get one serving for this

You will need:

- A single avocado (organic)
- A single ounce of goat cheese (use soft and fresh)
- 2 ounces of smoked salmon (wild-caught)
- 2 tablespoons of olive oil (use organic and make sure that it is extra virgin)
- The juice from a single lemon
- a pinch of salt (use celtic sea salt)

What you need to do:

1. Cut your avocado in two pieces and remove the pit.
2. In a food processor, add the rest of your ingredients until they have been chopped coarsely.
3. Place mixture inside your avocado.

Nutritional information:

- Calories-525
- Fat-48 grams
- Carbs-4 grams
- Protein-19 grams

Egg soup

You will need minutes for this

You will get one serving from this

What you need:

- A single cup and a half of chicken broth
- A half cube of chicken bouillon
- A single tablespoon of bacon fat
- 2 eggs (use large ones)
- A single teaspoon of chili garlic paste

What you need to do:

1. Get a pan and place it on your stove before setting your heat to medium-high.
2. Add the broth, fat, and bouillon cube.
3. Bring your broth to boiling and stir.
4. Add your paste and stir.
5. Turn off your stove.
6. Get a bowl.
7. Beat your eggs in the bowl before you pour it in the broth.
8. Stir well.
9. Let sit for a moment so that it will cook.

Nutritional information:

- Calories-289
- Fat-23.24 grams
- Carbs-2.92 grams
- Protein-15.3 grams

Queso soup

You will need 35 minutes for this

You will get 4 servings from this

What you need:

- A single tablespoon of taco seasoning
- A single pound of chicken breast
- A single tablespoon of avocado oil 3 cups of broth (use chicken)
- 2 cans Rotel that are ten ounces with green chiles (diced)
- 8 ounces of cream cheese
- Half of a cup of heavy cream

What you need to do:

1. Get a pot or a dutch oven that is cast iron.
2. Turn your heat to medium.
3. Heat the oil.
4. Stir your Rotel into the pot.
5. Stir the seasoning in the pot.
6. Cook for a single minute.
7. Add in the chicken.
8. Add in your broth.
9. Cover your pan.
10. You will need to simmer for 25 minutes.
11. Remove your chicken and then proceed to shred it.

12. Set the chicken to the side.
13. Stir in your heavy cream.
14. Stir in your cream cheese.
15. When the cheese has melted, put the chicken back in the pot.
16. Season with salt and pepper if you so choose.

Nutritional information:

- Calories-491
- Fat-37.6 grams
- Protein-33.1 grams
- Carbs-9.6 grams

Smoked salmon

You will need 20 minutes for this

You will get 6 servings from this

What you need:

- 7 ounces of salmon (smoked)
- The zest from half of a lemon)
- 8 ounces of cream cheese
- 4 tablespoons of dill (fresh)
- 5 and an additional 1/3 tablespoons of mayo
- 2 ounces of lettuce

What you need to do:

1. Cut your salmon into pieces that are small.
2. Combine all of your ingredients in a bowl.
3. Let it sit for 15 minutes.
4. This lets the flavors develop.
5. Place on a lettuce leaf.

Nutritional information:

- Calories-330
- Fat-26 grams
- Protein- 23 grams
- Carbs-3 grams

Butter shrimp

You will need 25 minutes for this

You will get 4 servings for this

You will need:

- A single pound of raw shrimp (it will need to be large, wild-caught and you will need to devein it and peel it)
- 3 tablespoons of water
- Half a dozen sprigs of oregano (it will need to be fresh)
- A single cup of ghee (you should go for grass-fed)
- A single bay leaf
- A single zest from a lemon

What you need to do:

1. Get yourself a pan.
2. Bring water to a boil. To do so, your heat should be high.
3. Reduce your heat to medium before whisking in the ghee.
4. Whisk constantly.
5. Your sauce should become smooth, and the texture should be even.
6. Add the rest of your ingredients except water and sprinkle with salt.

7. Stir, so the shrimp gets coated.
8. Lay them evenly in your pan.
9. Bring the liquid in the pan up to a light simmer. Your heat should now be medium-low.
10. Cook your shrimp for five minutes. Make sure it's cooked all the way through and pink.
11. Serve with a little sauce and dill.

Nutritional information:

- Calories-304
- Fat-27 grams
- Carbs-5 grams
- Protein- 13 grams

Baked salmon

You will need 15 minutes for this

You will get 4 servings from this

What you need for the Salmon:

- 2 pounds of salmon
- 4 tablespoons of pesto (green)

What you need for the sauce:

- A single cup of mayo
- Half of a cup of yogurt (make sure that it is full fat and Greek)
- 4 tablespoons of pesto (green)

What you need to do:

1. Place your salmon in a baking dish that is greased.
2. Be sure its skin side down.
3. Spread the pesto over the top.
4. Bake for half an hour at 400 degrees.
5. The fish should flake easily with a fork.
6. Stir all of the sauce ingredients together.

Nutritional information:

- Calories-1037
- Fat-90 grams
- Fiber-0 grams
- Protein-50 grams
- Carbs-3 grams

Tomato soup

You will need 15 minutes for this

You will get six servings from it

What you need:

- A stick of unsalted butter
- 8 ounces of cream cheese
- 5 cups of tomato puree (you will get this by blending fresh tomato chunks (minus the stems))
- One handful of basil leaves (fresh)
- If you like add salt and pepper for tasting

What you need to do:

1. Puree the tomatoes to get five cups (an estimate to help you is that this would be about 4 large tomatoes and around a pint of cherry tomatoes)
2. Get a saucepan.
3. Pour the puree into the pan.
4. Add the cream cheese and butter.
5. Heat to a simmer and cook until both the butter and cream cheese melt.
6. Pour the soup back into your blender.
7. Add your basil.
8. Be sure that you are venting the lid as this is a hot liquid.

9. Puree till smooth.

Nutritional information:

- Calories-287
- Fat-28 grams
- Carbs-6 grams
- Protein-3 grams
- Fiber-1 gram

Salad on the go

You will need 10 minutes for this

You will get a single serving from this

What you need:

- A single avocado
- A single ounce of bell peppers. For this recipe, you should use red.
- A single ounce of cherry tomatoes
- A single carrot
- ½ of a scallion (make sure that it is sliced)
- A single ounce of leafy greens
- 4 ounces of rotisserie chicken or salmon that has been smoked (wherever your preference lies)
- ¼ of a cup of mayo or olive oil (wherever your preference lies)

What you need to do:

1. Chop the vegetables or shred them.
2. Get a jar.
3. Put the leafy greens at the bottom.
4. Add the other ingredients in layers.
5. Add the chicken or salmon to the top.
6. Add the mayo or oil.

This is fun to play around with. You could use eggs or tuna; this is perfect for women with a busy lifestyle.

Nutritional information:

- Calories-1133
- Fat-84 grams
- Fiber-17 grams
- Protein-75 grams
- Carbs-11 grams

Salmon plate

You will need 5 minutes for this

You will get 2 servings from this

What you need:

- 2 avocados
- Salt and pepper if you like for flavor and taste
- ½ of a cup of mayo
- 7 ounces of smoked salmon

What you will need to do:

- Split your avocados in half.
- Remove the pit before scooping the rest out with a spoon.
- Cut the leftover avocado (what you scooped out. The good stuff not the pit) into pieces.
- Place the pieces on a plate.
- Add your salmon to the plate and a dollop of mayo.
- Sprinkle the salt and pepper over the top.

Nutritional information:

Per serving.

- Calories-1037
- Protein-65 grams
- Fat-82 grams
- Fiber-13 grams
- Carbs- 2 grams

Slaw bowl

You will need 15 minutes for this

You will get 4 servings from this

What you need:

- A single teaspoon of avocado oil
- A single pound of ground beef
- 2 teaspoons of toasted sesame oil
- A quarter of a cup of green onions
- 1 teaspoon of sea salt
- A quarter of a cup of black pepper
- 4 cups of shredded coleslaw mix
- 3 tablespoons of ginger (fresh)
- 4 minced garlic cloves
- A quarter cup of coconut aminos
- A quarter cup of green onions

What you need to do:

1. In a large saute pan, you will need to heat your avocado oil on a heat that has been set to medium-high.
2. Add ginger and garlic.
3. Saute for a minute.
4. The smell should be fragrant for you.
5. Add the beef and season.
6. Cook between seven and ten minutes. The meat should be browned at this point.

7. Reduce the heat to medium.
8. Add the coconut and coleslaw mix and stir.
9. Cover it and cook for five minutes.
10.   Remove from the heat and stir in your toppings (the sesame oil and onions)

Nutritional information:

One serving is 1 ½ cups (this would be the whole meal). If you have it with something else (like a side dish), it's one cup for a serving.

- Calories-457
- Fat-31 grams
- Protein-33 grams
- Carbs- 9 grams
- Fiber- 2 grams

Grilled steak

You will need 17 minutes for this

You will get around 6 servings to 8 servings with this

What you need for the sauce:

- A single clove of garlic
- A single tablespoon of oregano (fresh)
- ½ of a teaspoon of salt
- 4 tablespoons of oil (olive)
- ¼ of a teaspoon of pepper
- ¼ of a teaspoon of pepper flakes (red ones)
- A single tablespoon of lime juice (fresh)
- 3 diced avocados
- 3 tablespoons of vinegar (used red wine)

What you need for the meat:

- 2 pounds of flank steak
- Pepper for seasoning
- Salt for seasoning

What you need to do:

1. Heat a grill to medium-high heat or to 400 degrees.
2. Add all of the ingredients for the sauce to a food processor and blend until everything is smooth.

3. Get yourself a bowl.
4. Add the avocado and the sauce you blended.
5. Toss lightly, so it gets coated but not hard enough to crush the avocado.
6. Take a room temperature flank steak and season both sides with pepper and salt.
7. Place the steak on the grill and cook for a maximum of six minutes on each side and a minimum of four minutes.
8. Remove from your grill and let cool for a few minutes.
9. Slice the steak and drizzle the top with sauce or serve it on the side.

Nutritional information:

The serving size for this recipe is one steak (5 ounces) and sauce

- Calories-444
- Fat-32 grams
- Fiber-5 grams
- Protein-34 grams

Carbs-7 grams

Chapter 5: Dinner Recipes

Pork

You will need 35 minutes for this recipe

You will get 2 servings from this

What you need:

- A single pound of pork tenderloin
- A quarter cup of oil
- 3 medium shallots (chop them finely)

What you need to do:

1. Slice your pork into thick slices (go for about a half-inch thick).
2. Chop up your shallots before placing them on a plate.
3. Get a cast-iron skillet and warm up the oil
4. Press your pork into your shallots on both sides. Press firmly to make sure that they stick.
5. Place the slices of pork with shallots into the warm oil and then cook until it's done. The shallots may burn, but they will still be fine.
6. Make sure the pork is cooked through thoroughly.

Nutritional information:

- Calories-519
- Fat-36 grams
- Protein-46 grams
- Carbs-7 grams

Garlic shrimp

You will need 20 minutes for this

You will get 3 servings for this

What you need:

- 2 minced garlic cloves
- 2 whole garlic cloves
- The juice from half a lemon
- 2 tablespoons of oil (olive)
- 2 tablespoons of butter
- ¾ pounds of either small or medium shrimp (it needs to be both shelled and deveined)
- A quarter of a teaspoon of paprika
- A quarter of a teaspoon of pepper flakes (red ones)
- 2 tablespoons of parsley that is chopped.

What you have to do:

1. Sprinkle your shrimp with a teaspoon of salt (fine grain sea salt) and let it sit for ten minutes.
2. Get a skillet.
3. Heat the butter with olive oil over a heat that is medium-high.
4. Add the flakes and garlic.
5. Saute for half a minute.

6. Add your shrimp and cook until they have turned pink. This will take approximately two minutes. Stir constantly.
7. Add paprika and juice from the lemon.
8. Cook for another sixty seconds.

Nutritional information:
Per serving
- Calories-260
- Fat-18 grams
- Carbs-none
- Protein-24 protein

Pork Chop

You will need 40 minutes for this

You will get 6 servings for this

You will need:

- A dozen pork chop (boneless and thin cut)
- 2 cups of spinach (you should use baby spinach for this)
- 4 cloves of garlic
- A dozen slices provolone cheese

You will need to do the following things:

1. Preheat your oven to a temperature of 350.
2. Press the garlic cloves using a garlic press. The cloves should go through the press and into a small bowl.
3. Spread the garlic that you have made onto one side of the pork chops.
4. Flip half a dozen chops while making sure the garlic side is down.
5. You should do this on a baking sheet that is rimmed.
6. Divide your spinach between the half dozen chops.
7. Fold cheese slices in half.
8. Put them on top of the spinach.

9. Put a second pork chop on top of the first set, but this time make sure that the garlic side is up.
10.   Bake for 20 minutes.
11.   Cover each chop with another piece of cheese.
12.   Bake another 15 minutes.
13.   Your meat meter should be at 160 degrees when you check with a thermometer.

Nutritional information:

- Calories-436
- Fat-25 grams
- Carbs-2 grams
- Protein-47 grams

Citrus egg salad

You will need 10 minutes for this

You get 3 servings from this

What you need:

- Half a dozen eggs (6)
- A single teaspoon of mustard (go with Dijon)
- 2 tablespoons of mayo
- A single teaspoon of lemon juice

What you need to do:

1. Place the eggs gently in a medium saucepan.
2. Add cold water until your eggs are covered by an inch.
3. Bring to a boil.
4. You should do this for ten minutes. Remove from your heat and cool. Peel your eggs under running water that is cold .
5. Put your eggs in a food processor. Pulse until they are chopped.
6. Stir in condiments and juice.

Nutritional information:

- Calories-222
- Fat-19 grams
- Protein-13 grams
- Carbs-1 gram

Chowder

You will need 40 minutes

You will get 4 servings from this

You will need:

- A single tablespoon of butter
- 5 minced garlic cloves
- An entire head of cauliflower (cut it into florets that are small)
- Half of a teaspoon of oregano (use dried)
- Half a cup of carrots that have been diced
- Half a cup of onions that have been diced
- A cup and a half of broth (use vegetable)
- A quarter cup of cream cheese

What you need to do:

1. Get a soup pot.
2. Heat your butter.
3. Add garlic and onions.
4. Saute for a few moments.
5. Add the rest of the ingredients to the pot.
6. Bring to a boil.
7. Slow the heat and put it on a simmer.
8. Cook for 15 minutes.
9. Shut off the flame.
10. Use a hand blender to blend the soup partly in the pot.
11. Switch the flame back on.
12. Add a cup of broth.

13.   Add the cream cheese.

14.   Simmer for 10 minutes and switch off the flame again.

Nutritional information:

Per serving

- Calories-143
- Fat-8.4 grams
- Carbs-15.2 grams
- Protein-4.5 grams

Avocado salad

You need 10 minutes for this

You get one serving from this

What you need:

• 3 ounces of cooked and shredded chicken breast
• A single stalk of celery
• A single tablespoon of diced red onions
• A third of a cup of sour cream
• A single avocado (go with a medium)

What you need to do:

1. Cook the chicken on low heat until it is fully cooked.
2. Shred it using forks.
3. Get a bowl.
4. Place your celery, chicken, and onion inside to combine.
5. Cut your avocado and put your avocado.
6. Scoop some of the avocado out before putting it in the bowl.
7. Add the sour cream.
8. Toss everything well.
9. Put the mix back in the avocado halves.

Nutritional information:

- Calories-570
- Protein-29 grams
- Fat-45 grams
- Carbs-5 grams

Tex plate

You will need 20 minutes for this

You will get 6 servings for this

You will need:

- ⅔ of a pound of ground beef
- 4 tablespoons of olive oil
- 2 tablespoons of water. It needs to be cold.
- A single tablespoon of seasoning (go with tex mex on this one)
- A single ounce of sliced pepper jack cheese (for a kick)
- 2 avocados
- 2 tablespoons of jalapenos (they need to be pickled)
- A third of a cup of mayo
- 2 ounces arugula lettuce

What you need to do:

1. Mix the water, meat, and seasoning.
2. Form one burger per serving.
3. Brush half of the olive oil that you have around each burger that you have.
4. Fry them for four minutes on each side. The burger should be light pink or cooked entirely through.
5. Place your burger on a plate with all the other vegetables and cheese.

6.   Drizzle the oil over the top of everything.

Nutritional information:

- Calories-1067
- Fiber-15 grams
- Carbs- 7 grams
- Protein-39 grams
- Fat-95 grams

Eggs and tuna

You will need 10 minutes for this

You will get 2 servings of this

What you need:

- 2 tablespoons of olive oil
- 2 tablespoons of capers that are small
- 2 ounces of tomatoes (cherry)
- 2 ounces lettuce
- 4 ounces of tuna (it needs to be in olive oil and drained)
- Half of a lemon you want the zest and juice from it
- A third of a cup of celery stalks that have been chopped
- Half a cup of mayo
- Half of a red onion
- A single teaspoon of mustard (use dijon)

For your eggs:

- 4 ounces
- 2 teaspoons of vinegar (white wine vinegar)
- A single teaspoon of salt

What you need to do for this:

1.   Mix your tuna with the other ingredients on the first list. Don't mix the lettuce or tomatoes, however.

2. Bring water in a pot to a light boil.

3. Add in the vinegar and salt before stirring the water. You should be making a swirl with your spoon.

4. Crack the egg into the water while it's moving.

5. Do this one at a time.

6. Let it simmer for three minutes.

7. Remove from your water using a spoon that is slotted.

8. Use the lettuce and tomatoes when you're ready to eat and pour the olive oil over the top.

Nutritional information:

- Calories-765
- Fiber-3 grams
- Carbs-6 grams
- Fat- 69 grams
- Protein-29 grams

Fried chicken

You will need 15 minutes for this

You will get 2 servings

You will need:

- 10 ounces of chicken thighs that are boneless
- 9 ounces of broccoli
- 3 and a half ounces of butter

What you need to do:

1. Rinse the broccoli.
2. Trim the broccoli as well.
3. Cut the broccoli into small pieces. This will include the stem.
4. Heat up a good part of the butter in a pan for frying.
5. Season your chicken with pepper and salt if you like.
6. Fry it over a heat that is medium for 5 minutes per side. It should be cooked through.
7. Add another helping of the butter and put the broccoli in the same pan you have been using and fry the broccoli for two minutes.
8. Season more (if you need to. If you don't, then leave it as is.), and then when you plate it serve it with the rest of the butter that you haven't used.

Nutritional information:

- Calories-733
- Fiber- 3 grams
- Fat-66 grams
- Carbs-5 grams
- Protein-29 grams

Ground beef plate

You will need 15 minutes for this

You will get 2 servings from this

You will need:

- 10 ounces of ground beef
- 3 and a half ounces of butter
- 9 ounces of green beans that are fresh

What you will need to do:

- Rinse your green beans.
- Trim them.
- Heat up part of your butter in a pan for frying.
- Brown your ground beef on a heat that is high until it is almost done.
- Lower your heat and on the opposite side of the pan (next to the meat), add another portion of butter.
- Fry your green beans for five minutes.
- Stir your ground beef.
- Season beans with salt and pepper if you wish.
- Plate everything and serve with the rest of the butter.

Nutritional information:

- Calories-694
- Fat-60 grams
- Fiber-3 grams
- Carbs-5 grams
- Protein-32 grams

Mac n cheese

You will need 4 minutes for this

You will get one serving from this

What you need:

- A single ounce of shredded cheddar cheese
- A single tablespoon of heavy cream
- ¾ of a cup of florets of cauliflower that are frozen

What you need to do:

1. Get a microwavable dish that has a lid.
2. Microwave it covered for a minute.
3. Remove and chop the cauliflower. The pieces should be small.
4. Microwave for another 50 seconds and add the cheese.
5. Microwave 10 seconds.
6. Stir and stir in the heavy cream. This will form a sauce.

Nutritional information:

- Calories-191
- Fat-14.9
- Fiber-2
- Carbs-4.8
- Protein-9.4

Chicken with sauce

You will need 35 minutes for this

You will get 4 servings from this

You will need:

- 2 tablespoons of olive oil
- A single cup of keto dressing (use a keto honey mustard dressing)
- 4 chicken breasts that are skinless and boneless

You will need to do the following:

1. Combine the chicken and half of your dressing into a bowl.
2. Toss the chicken so it can get coated.
3. You will need to let it marinate in the fridge for an hour. If you have more time, you can do it up to 24 hours.
4. Preheat your oven to 350.
5. Heat the oil in a skillet that is oven-proof.
6. The heat should be medium-high.
7. When your pan is hot, you can add the chicken.
8. You will pan sear the chicken and brown it on both sides.
9. This will be 4 minutes on each side.
10. Pour the rest of the dressing on the chicken.
11. Transfer the skillet to the oven.

12.   Bake 20 minutes.

13.   The chicken should be cooked all the way through, but if not, cook longer.

Nutritional information:

- Calories-242
- Fat-9.5 grams
- Protein-34 grams
- Carbs-1 gram

Chili pot

You will need an hour and five minutes for this

You will get 6 servings from this

What you will need:

- A single tablespoon and a half of avocado oil
- 2 pounds of pork shoulder (be sure to cut it into half a dozen pieces (6))
- A single cup and a half of salsa verde (herdez is a good brand)
- A single cup of broth (chicken broth)

What you need to do:

1. Rub your pork pieces with pepper and salt.
2. You will need an instant pot for this recipe.
3. Select the saute button.
4. Add the oil to the inner pot of the instant pot.
5. When the pot is hot, sear the pork pieces on all of the sides. Each side will take four minutes per side until they have browned.
6. In a bowl, combine your broth and salsa verde.
7. Stir.
8. Pour the mix over the pork.
9. Close and lock the lid of the instant pot.
10. Turn your pressure release handle to sealing.
11. Select pressure cooker manual on high pressure.
12. Set your timer for forty minutes.

13.   It will take a bit to start, but it will beep and then begin to countdown.

14.   Once your cooking time is done, you need to let the pressure naturally release for 10 minutes. This means let the pot sit for those minutes.

15.   Quick-release the remaining pressure. A good trick is to use a spoon made of wood to press the release handle to vent. You should keep your hands and face away from the steam, so you don't hurt yourself.

16.   When the pressure is released, remove your lid.

17.   Remove the pork and place on a plate.

18.   Shred the pork.

19.   Add the shredded pork back into the sauce that is still in the pot.

20.   Stir so that it can combine.

Nutritional information:

- Calories-342
- Fat-22 grams
- Fiber-2 grams
- Carbs-4 grams
- Protein-32 grams

Scallops

You will need 25 minutes for this

You will need 4 servings for this

You will need:

- 8 bacon slices that are cut in half (make sure that they are cut crosswise)
- 16 sea scallops
- Olive oil
- Toothpicks for the scallops

The steps you need to follow:

1. Preheat your oven to 425.
2. Pat your scallops with a paper towel, so they dry.
3. Remove any side muscles from the scallops.
4. Wrap a scallop in one of the bacon halves and stick a toothpick in it.
5. Repeat with the other 15 scallops.
6. Pour your olive oil over the scallops, and if you want to season them with salt and pepper. If you choose to do this, make sure that you are using kosher salt.
7. Arrange your scallops in a layer on a baking sheet that is prepared. Make sure that they are in a single layer.
8. You need to leave space between them, so make sure to do so.

9.   Bake fifteen minutes. The scallops should be tender and look opaque while your bacon should be cooked through.
10.   Make sure that they are hot when you serve them.

Nutritional information:

- Calories-224
- Fat-17 grams
- Carbs- 2 grams
- Protein-12 grams

Chicken casserole

You're going to need 25 minutes

You will get 8 servings out of this

You will need:

- 16 ounces of salsa
- 3 cups of shredded chicken
- 8 ounces of softened cream cheese
- 8 ounces of shredded cheese (use cheddar)
- ¾ of a teaspoon of chipotle pepper (ground)

What you need to do:

1. Preheat your oven to 400.
2. Grease a baking dish that is 9 by 13.
3. Get a bowl.
4. Combine all of the ingredients but only half of the cheese and half a teaspoon of pepper.
5. Mix it well.
6. Put the mix in the baking dish.
7. Top the dish with the leftover cheese and pepper.
8. Bake 20 minutes. It should be bubbly and hot.

Nutritional information:

- Calories- 319
- Fat-25 grams
- Fiber-1 gram
- Carbs-5 grams
- Protein-17 grams

Shrimp noodles

You will need 15 minutes for this

You will get 2 servings from this

You will need:

- A single tablespoon of olive oil
- The zest and juice from an entire lemon
- 2 zucchini that are medium in size
- 3 to 4 minced garlic cloves
- ¾ pounds of shrimp that are medium in size as well as peeled and deveined
- Fresh parsley that is chopped

What you will need to do:

1. With the zucchini, spiralize it on a setting of medium.
2. Set the spiralized veggie aside.
3. Get a skillet and put the heat to medium.
4. Add the lemon zest and juice along with olive oil to the pan.
5. Once the pan is warm, you can add the shrimp.
6. Cook the shrimp for a single minute on each side.
7. Add garlic and cook for a minute, making sure to stir.

8.   Add the noodles (veggie noodles) and stir for 3 minutes. This is going to warm them up and cook them. If it helps use tongs.
9.   Sprinkle with your parsley.
10.   Serve right away.

Nutritional information:

- Calories-280

Tuna patties

You're going to need 15 minutes for this

You will get 6 servings for this

What you will need:

- One half of a cup of shredded cheese
- 2 eggs
- 4 ounces of pork rinds (we need them ground up into crumbs)
- 2 tablespoons of pico de gallo
- 2 cans of tuna that has been packed in water and 5 ounces each

What you will need to do:

1. Open your tuna and drain it.
2. Pulse your rinds in a food processor, so they become crumbs.
3. Get a bowl.
4. Mix all the ingredients until they have combined fully.
5. Separate the mixture so that you have six parts that you can make into patties.
6. Roll into six patties.
7. Fry in coconut oil for a few minutes on each of the sides.
8. When done, they should be golden brown.
9. Serve while they are warm.

Nutritional information:

One patty is one serving

- Calories-205
- Carbs-1.4 grams
- Fat- 11.5 grams
- Protein-22.6 grams

Meatballs

You will need 20 minutes for this

You will get 3 servings from this

You will need the following:

- A single teaspoon of garlic powder
- 3.5 ounces of mozzarella cheese
- 1.1 pounds of ground beef
- 3 tablespoons of parmesan cheese

What you will need to do:

1. Cut your cheese into cubes. Ideally, you want a single centimeter by a single centimeter.
2. Mix your dry ingredients with your ground beef.
3. Wrap the cubes that you made in the meat. You should get at least nine balls.
4. Pan-fry the meatballs.
5. Make sure to have a lid to capture the heat.
6. Make sure the cheese doesn't spill.

Nutritional information:

- Calories-444
- Fat-28 grams
- Protein-46 grams
- Carbs-2 grams

Chicken breasts

You will need a half-hour for this recipe

You're going to get 6 servings from this

What you need:

- A quarter of a cup of Greek yogurt
- Half of a cup of shredded mozzarella cheese
- 2 tablespoons of olive oil
- A pound and a half of chicken breasts. They need to be four-ounce portions
- A quarter cup of spinach. Frozen and drained, it should also be tightly packed.
- Half of a cup of thinly sliced artichoke hearts
- 4 ounces of softened cream cheese
- Half a teaspoon of divided salt
- A quarter of a teaspoon of divided pepper

What you need to do:

1. Pound your chicken breast to a single inch thick.
2. Use a sharp knife carefully and cut each breast down the middle. Do not cut all of the way. You are making a pocket.
3. Sprinkle the breasts with a quarter teaspoon of salt.
4. Sprinkle then with an eighth of a teaspoon of pepper.
5. Get a bowl.

6.   Combine everything except your oil and mix it thoroughly. You need the ingredients to combine thoroughly.

7.   Fill each breast with the mixture.

8.   Get a large skillet.

9.   Turn the heat to medium.

10.   In the skillet, add your oil and breasts.

11.   Cover the skillet and cook for 8 minutes on each side.

12.   Your chicken should reach 165 degrees when you check it with a meat thermometer.

13.   When it's the last few minutes of your cooking, add any leftover filling to the skillet, so it heats up.

14.   Server your chicken with cauliflower rice.

Nutritional information:

- Calories-288
- Fat-17 grams
- Protein-28 grams
- Carbs-2 grams

Cream cheese rollups

You will need 10 minutes for this

You will get 15 servings from this

You will need:

- 7 and a half teaspoons of chopped banana peppers
- 1.25 ounces of cream cheese
- 7 and a half teaspoons chopped red peppers
- 15 slices of salami

You will need to do the following:

1. Spread half a teaspoon of your cream cheese on each slice of your salami.
2. Spoon a single teaspoon of your red pepper on 5 slices of salami.
3. For the last five slices, you want to place half a teaspoon of each pepper onto the meat.
4. Fold each slice of meat over, so it looks like a taco.
5. If you need to keep it closed, use a toothpick.

Nutritional information:

One serving= one rollup

- Calories-50
- Fat-4.04 grams
- Fiber-0.06 grams
- Carbs-0.61 grams
- Protein-2.88 grams

Cheesy Quiche

You will need 35 minutes for this

You will get 9 servings from this

You will need:

- 7 eggs
- Half a cup of heavy cream
- 12 ounces of chopped broccoli
- 2 tablespoons of almond flour
- A cup and a third of cheese. (use sharp cheddar)
- Half of a cup of chopped red onions
- Half a teaspoon of ground mustard

What you need to do:

1. Preheat your oven to 350.
2. Spray a muffin tin (a small one) with a non-stick cooking spray.
3. Lightly flour the bottom.
4. Get a bowl.
5. Whisk your ingredients except the cheese, onions, and broccoli.
6. Stir in the broccoli cheese and onions.
7. Pour the mix into the baking tin.
8. Bake 40 minutes.
9. A knife should come out clean.

Nutritional information:

- Calories-183
- Fat-14.04 grams
- Fiber-0.58 grams
- Protein-9.06 grams
- Carbs-2.79 grams

Dinner box

You will need 15 minutes for this

You will get one serving from this

You will need:

- 2 tablespoons of almonds that are raw
- A single hard-boiled large egg
- A quarter cup of cherry tomatoes
- 2 ounces of turkey breast that are thinly sliced
- 4 pita bites crackers
- A single ounce of cubed and sharp cheddar cheese

What you need to do:

1. Get a meal prep container or a piece of tupperware that resembles one.
2. Place the ingredients in the container in any way you like.

Nutritional information:

- Calories-382
- Protein-23 grams
- Carbs-16 grams
- Fiber-3 grams
- Fat-25 grams

Elegant taco salad

You will need 20 minutes for this

You will get 6 servings from this

You will need:

- 8 ounces of chopped romaine lettuce
- A third of a cup of salsa
- A third of a cup of sour cream
- A single cubed medium avocado
- A single pound of ground beef
- A single teaspoon of avocado oil
- A cup and a third of halved grape tomatoes
- Half a cup of chopped green onions
- ¾ of a cup of shredded cheddar cheese
- 2 tablespoons of taco seasoning

You will need to do the following:

1. Get a skillet.
2. Heat your oil in the skillet at a heat that is high.
3. Add your beef.
4. Stir fry while making sure that you are breaking the pieces up.
5. You will need to stir fry for 10 minutes.
6. The beef should be browned, and the moisture should be evaporated.
7. Stir in the seasoning into the beef. Make sure it has combined well.

8.   Get a bowl.

9.   Place all of the remaining ingredients in the bowl.

10.   Add the beef.

11.   Toss it all together.

Nutritional information:

Serving size is ⅙ of the recipe

- Calories-332
- Fat-25 grams
- Protein-20 grams
- Carbs-9 grams
- Fiber-4 grams

Loaded casserole

You will need an hour for this

You will get 8 servings from this

You will need:

- A single cup of cheddar cheese that is sharp
- A single head of cauliflower that is large and cut into florets
- A single cup of shredded cheese (use colby and monterey jack)
- 8 slices of bacon that has been fried crispy
- 6 tablespoons of chives that are fresh, chopped and divided
- Half of a cup of sour cream
- A single tablespoon of ranch seasoning
- Half a cup of mayo

You will need to do the following:

1. Preheat your oven to 370.
2. Get a baking dish that is 13 by 9 and spray with a non-stick cooking spray.
3. Get a large skillet.
4. Fry the bacon until it becomes crispy.
5. Crumble it and place to the side.
6. Steam the cauliflower for 20 minutes, as this will make it tender.
7. Get a bowl.

8.   Combine the seasoning, mayo, and sour cream before adding the cauliflower, 3 tablespoons of chives, half of your bacon, and a cup of the cheddar.

9.   Mix it all well.

10.   Pour the mixture into the baking dish.

11.   Top it with colby and monterey jack cheese.

12.   Top that with the other half of the bacon.

13.   Cover the dish with foil.

14.   Bake for 20 minutes.

15.   Take the foil off.

16.   Bake for another 10 minutes. Your cheese should be bubbly, and the color should be turning brown.

17.   Top with the other half of the chives.

Nutritional information:

3/4 cup makes one serving

- Calories-297
- Protein 11.4 grams
- Fat-26.6 grams
- Fiber-0.5 grams
- Carbs-3 grams

Tomato avocados

You will need 15 minutes for this

You will get 4 servings from this

You will need:

- 2 bacon slices
- A quarter teaspoon of garlic powder
- A single teaspoon of lime juice
- Half of a cup of halved grape tomatoes
- 2 avocados that are medium in size
- Half a cup of chopped romaine lettuce

What you will need:

1. Get a skillet.
2. Place your bacon inside the skillet while the pan is still cold.
3. Cook bacon on low or medium-low heat. You want the edges to curl.
4. Flip the bacon.
5. Continue cooking until it becomes crispy and golden in color.
6. This can take 5 minutes or longer.
7. Drain on paper towels.
8. Slice your avocados in half.
9. Leave half of the halves alone but scoop the middle out of the other halves.
10. Put it in a bowl.

11.   Mash the avocados that you put in the bowl and add in the rest of your ingredients besides the bacon.

12.   When the bacon has cooled, chop it up.

13.   Add to the bowl.

14.   Scoop the mixture in the bowl into all of the halves

Nutritional information:

One serving is half an avocado with filing

- Calories-189
- Fat-16 grams
- Fiber-7 grams
- Carbs-10 grams
- Protein-4 grams

Egg pie

You will need 40 minutes for this

You will get 6 servings from this

You will need:

- 2 slices of diced bacon
- A single spring of finely sliced onion
- 8 medium eggs
- 4.2 fluid ounces of full-fat milk
- 3 and a half ounces of shredded cheese

You will need to do the following:

1. Get a bowl.
2. Whisk your milk and eggs with a fork.
3. Add everything else to the bowl and stir gently.
4. Get a 20 by 8 baking dish and grease it and line it with baking paper.
5. Bake at 350 degrees for a half-hour.

Nutritional information:

- Calories-201
- Fat-17.7 grams
- Carbs-1.4 grams
- Protein-18 grams

Turkey Roll

You will need five minutes for this

You can get two servings out of this

You will need:

- A sliced avocado
- 2 ounces of lettuce
- 4 tablespoons of olive oil
- 3 ounces of cream cheese
- 6 ounces of turkey (use deli turkey)
- Salt and pepper for some flavor or taste if you like

What you will need to do:

1. Roll your turkey.
2. Arrange the vegetables around the turkey on a plate to make it look pleasing.
3. Arrange the cream cheese on the plate.
4. Drizzle olive oil over your vegetables and season with pepper and salt if need be.

Nutritional information:

- Calories-660
- Fat-60 grams
- Fiber-7 grams
- Protein-22 grams
- Carbs-7 grams

Roast beef rolls

You will need 5 minutes for this

You will get 2 servings from this

You will need:

- A single avocado
- A single scallion
- A half of a cup of mayo
- 5 ounces of cheese (use cheddar)
- Half a dozen radishes (six)
- 2 ounces of lettuce
- 2 tablespoons of olive oil
- 7 ounces of roast beef (use deli roast beef)
- A single tablespoon of mustard (use dijon)
- Salt and pepper for flavor

What you will need to do:

1. Roll the roast beef and set it on the plate, leaving room for the cheese and vegetables to go in between.
2. Put the sauces in the middle for dipping.
3. When you are ready to eat it, you can serve it with the lettuce and the olive oil over the top of the veggies for a great flavor.

Nutritional information:

- Calories-1071
- Fat-98 grams
- Fiber-8 grams
- Protein-38 grams
- Carbs-6 grams

Shrimp eggs

You will need 10 minutes to prepare

You will get 4 servings from this

What you need:

- Fresh dill
- A quarter cup of mayo
- A single teaspoon of tabasco
- A pinch of salt (use herbal salt)
- 4 eggs
- 8 cooked shrimp

What you will need:

1. Get a pot and begin boiling your eggs.
2. Boil the eggs for a minimum of eight minutes and a maximum of ten.
3. Remove the eggs from your pot.
4. Give them an ice bath for a few minutes.
5. Peel your eggs.
6. Split the eggs in half before scooping out the yolks.
7. Get yourself a bowl.
8. Mask the yolks in the bowl and add in your mayo, tabasco sauce, and salt.
9. Add the mixture to the eggs and place a shrimp on top.

Nutritional information:

- Calories-163
- Carbs-0.5 grams
- Protein-7 grams
- Fat-15 grams

Chapter 6: Snack Recipes

Chips

You only need five minutes to make this!

You will get four servings from this

What you need for the chip:

- A bag of pork rinds (take note that whatever bag you choose will change the nutrition information at the end of the recipe)
- Oil spray (make sure its avocado)

What you need for the coating:

- A single tablespoon of paprika
- ½ of a tablespoon of cayenne pepper for a little bit of a kick
- ½ of a tablespoon of onion powder
- ¼ of a cup of nutritional yeast
- ½ garlic powder

What you need to do:

1. Add the coating ingredients to a spice grinder and blend until everything becomes smooth.
2. Spray your pork rinds with oil as it will make the coating stick better.

3. Transfer the rinds to a plastic bag and pour the toppings in before you begin to shake it.

Nutritional information:

- Calories-97
- Fat-2.7 grams
- Carbs-2 grams
- Fiber- 1 gram
- Protein-14 grams

Pickle time!

This will only take you five minutes

You can get up to four servings from this

What you need:

- A single can of tuna (go for a version that is light flaked)
- ¼ of a cup of mayo (it needs to be sugar-free if you can get it and a light version)
- A single tablespoon of dill
- 5 or 6 pickles depending on what you need

What you need to do:

1. Cut your pickles in half so that they are lengthwise.
2. Seed your pickles.
3. Drain the tuna and then mix the dill, mayo, and tuna in a bowl before mixing.
4. Spoon the tuna mix onto the pickle.

Nutritional information:

A serving size here is based on if you used six pickles.
Another note is that the nutritional information will change depending on what mayo you choose here.

- Calories-47.1
- Fiber-1.4 grams
- Protein 6.01 grams
- Carbs- 3.6 grams
- Fat-0.6

Hard-boiled eggs

You will need about 20 minutes to cook them and then time to cool them

You will be able to get twelve servings from this

What you need:

- A dozen eggs

What you need to do:

1. Get a pot that is big enough to hold the eggs.
2. Place six of the eggs in the pot.
3. Cover the eggs with cool water by an inch.
4. Cover your pan with a lid and bring your water to boiling.
5. Boil water in the pot for six minutes over medium-high heat
6. If you want them firmer, let them stay in the pot a little longer.
7. Repeat for the other six.

This is perfect for taking on the go and makes a quick protein-packed snack.

Nutritional information:

This is based upon two eggs.

- Calories-156
- Carbs-1 gram
- Fiber-o grams
- Fat-10.6 grams
- Protein-12.6 grams

Zingy crackers

You will need 25 minutes for this

You will get 16 pieces

You will need:

- A single pound cheddar cheese (sliced)
- 4 sliced jalapeno peppers (use sliced)

What you will need to do:

1. Heat oven to 425 and then line your baking sheet with parchment
2. Cut your cheese slices. They need to be 11/2 inch squares.
3. Arrange them on the baking sheet with at least an inch between them and then place a slice of jalapeno on top.
4. You will then place them in the oven and bake for a dozen minutes (12) .
5. You will know they are done when they are firm and light brown.
6. Remove and let them cool.
7. If stored in an airtight container, they will last two days.

Nutritional information:

- Calories-106
- Protein-7 grams
- Carbs-1 gram
- Fiber-0.3 grams
- Fat-9 grams

Pinwheel Delight

You will need ten minutes for this

You will get 20 pieces from this

What you need:

- A single block of cream cheese (8 ounces)
- 10 slices of salami (genoa) and pepperoni
- 4 tablespoons of pickles (make sure they are finely diced)

What you need to do:

1. Have your cream cheese brought to room temperature.
2. Whip the cream cheese until it becomes fluffy.
3. Spread your cream cheese in a rectangle that is a quarter-inch thick. Do this on a large piece of plastic wrap.
4. Place your pickles over cream cheese
5. Place the salami over the cream cheese in layers that are overlapping so that each cream cheese layer is covered.
6. Place another layer of wrap over the layer of salami and press down. Be gentle.
7. Flip your whole rectangle over so that the bottom cream cheese layer is now facing the top instead.
8. Peel back your plastic wrap off very carefully from the top cream cheese layer.

9. You should begin rolling this into a log shape, slowly removing the bottom layer of your plastic wrap as you go along.
10. Place the pinwheel in a tight plastic wrap.
11. Place in the fridge overnight or if you can't wait at least four hours.
12. Slice however thick you want it.

Nutritional information:

- Calories- 47
- Fat-4.2 grams
- Protein-1 gram
- Carbs-0.8 grams

This is based on a single pinwheel

Zesty olives

You will need 10 minutes for this recipe

You will get up to 6 servings out of this maximum and 4 at a minimum

What you need:

- 1/4 of a cup of oil (make sure that it is extra virgin olive oil)
- 1/4 of a teaspoon of pepper flakes (red and crushed)
- A single thinly sliced garlic clove
- A single tablespoon of lemon juice
- A single strip of zest from a lemon
- A single cup of olives (make sure that they are castelvetrano)
- 2 sprigs of thyme (make sure it's fresh)
- A single tablespoon of orange juice
- A single strip of zest from an orange

What you need to do:

1. Get a saucepan.
2. Heat your oil over a heat that is medium-high.
3. Add zest, thyme, garlic, and zest in and cook it.
4. Be sure that you stir occasionally.
5. Cook for a few minutes, and you will notice that the garlic is golden.

6. You will then need to stir in the olives and cook them as well.
7. Stir them as they cook but only cook for two minutes. You want them to be warmed.
8. Turn off your heat.
9. Stir in your juice.
10.   Place in a dish.

Nutritional information:

- Calories-180
- Fat- 20 grams
- Carbs- 2 grams

Deviled Eggs Keto Style!

This takes 10 minutes
You can get 20 deviled eggs here

What you need:

- 10 eggs (hardboiled of course)
- 10 large eggs, hardboiled
- A single avocado (make sure it is ripe)
- A single lemon (you will need to juice this)
- A single tablespoon of mustard (use Dijon)
- Paprika (use smoked)

What you need to do:

1. Slice your eggs in half and take out the yolks.
2. Combine your yolks, avocado, and lemon juice in a bowl and stir thoroughly.
3. Spoon the mixture into the egg halves.
4. Sprinkle the top with paprika.

Nutritional information:

- Calories-50
- Fat-4 grams
- Fiber-1 gram
- Protein- 3 grams
- Carbs- 1 gram

Cucumber time

You will need 5 minutes for this

You will get one serving from this

What you will need:

- A single cup of cucumbers (make sure they are sliced)
- 10 olived (kalamata olives. Use large ones)

What you need to do:

1. Mix them together in a bowl, and there you go!

Nutritional information:

- Calories-71
- Fiber-2.3 grams
- Carbs-5 grams
- Fat-4.8 grams
- Protein-1.29 grams

Nutty Yogurt

This will take 5 minutes

It will give you one serving

What you need:

- 2 ounces of yogurt (use whole milk greek yogurt)
- 1/2 of a teaspoon of cinnamon
- 1 tablespoon of walnuts (chopped)

What you need to do:

1. Place the yogurt in a dish.
2. Add the walnuts.
3. Add the cinnamon.

Nutritional information:

- Calories-160
- Fiber-0.5 grams
- Fat-12.5 grams
- Protein-8 grams
- Carbs-6 grams

Let's Get Crabby!

You will need 10 minutes for this

You can get 4 servings from this

What you need:

- A single avocado (make sure that it is ripe)
- 3 tablespoons of juice from a lemon.
- 2 tablespoons of chives (chopped)
- 1/2 of a pound of crab meat (lump)
- 1 teaspoon of mustard (use dijon)

What you need to do:

1. Put your avocados.
2. Peel them next.
3. Cut into chunks a half-inch thick.
4. Place them in a bowl.
5. Add a tablespoon of your juice.
6. In a separate bowl, add your other ingredients except the meat and whisk it together.
7. Add the meat and toss the ingredients.
8. Do the same for the last three servings.

Nutritional information:

- Calories-150
- Fat-8 grams
- Protein-15 grams
- Carbs-5 grams
- Fiber-3 grams

Cream And Berries

You will need 5 minutes to prepare this

You will get one serving from this

What you need:

- A quarter of a cup of berries (raspberries are best)
- A single cup of whipping cream

What you need to do:

1. Place the whipping cream on the bottom of your bowl.
2. Place your berries on top.

Nutritional information:

- Calories-230
- Fat-21.5 grams
- Protein-2 grams
- Fiber- 4 grams
- Carbs-5.1 grams

Let's go boating

You will need 5 minutes for this

You will get one serving out of this

What you need:

- A single celery stalk
- 2 tablespoons of peanut butter
- Chia seeds for the top if you desire to do so (it will give you a bit of omega-3s)

What you will need to do:

1. Cut the stalk into pieces after making sure that it is clean.
2. Place the peanut butter on top.
3. If you have chosen to use chia seeds, add them as well.

Nutritional information:

- Calories-225
- Fat-18.3 grams
- Fiber-4.6 grams
- Protein-9.3 grams
- Carbs-9.8 grams

Guacamole break

You will need five minutes for this

You will get a single serving from this

What you need:

- Half a cup of guacamole
- Half of a cucumber

What you need to do:

1. Cut the cucumber into slices after cleaning it.
2. Serve with the guacamole.

Nutritional information:

- Calories- 233
- Fat-19.9 grams
- Fiber-7.7 grams
- Carbs-14.9 grams
- Protein-3.2 grams

Creamy Dream

You will need five minutes for this

You will get one serving with this

What you need:

- 2 tablespoons almond butter (go with creamy it will mix better)
- A single teaspoon of flax seeds
- 2 teaspoons of pumpkin seeds
- A single teaspoon of sunflower seeds
- A single teaspoon of chia seeds

What you need to do:

1. Get a bowl.
2. Mix all the ingredients together.

The protein that you will get along with the fiber and fat should work to keep you full for longer.

Nutritional information:

- Calories-262
- Fat-21 grams
- Carbs-11.6 grams
- Protein-11 grams
- Fiber-7.8 grams

Creamy boat

You will need five minutes for this

You will get 2 servings from this

What you will need:

- 2 stalks of celery
- 2 tablespoons of cream cheese

What you need to do:

1. Clean the celery and cut it into pieces.
2. Place the pieces on a plate before adding cream cheese to them.
3. Repeat this process if necessary.

Nutritional information:

- Calories-113
- Fat-10.1 grams
- Fiber-1.3 grams
- Carbs-4 grams
- Protein-2.3 grams

Tomato Attack!

You will need 5 minutes for this

You will get one serving from this

What you need:

- 2 tablespoons of seeds (go with pumpkin on this one)
- Half a cup of cottage cheese (make sure it's full fat)
- A single teaspoon of olive oil
- 5 cherry tomato halves

What you need to do:

1. Place the halves on a plate in any formation, but a flower or a pattern that will leave the middle open for the cottage cheese is best.
2. The pumpkin seeds will make a great topping for the cottage cheese.

If you choose to add other vegetables like bell peppers, it will change the nutritional value, so be aware of this.

Nutritional information:

- Calories-201
- fat- 10.9 grams
- Protein-14.2 grams
- Fiber-2.5 grams
- Carbs-7.9 grams

Kabobs

You will need 5 minutes for this

You will get one serving out of this

What you need:

- A single ounce of salami (try to get a high quality if you can such as from a deli)
- A single ounce of cheese (your choice but you can have fun mixing and matching)

What you need to do:

1. Get a kabob stick and begin placing the cheese and meat upon it.
2. When you done, it's ready to be enjoyed.

Nutritional information:

- Calories-215
- Fat-16.5 grams
- Protein-14.8 grams
- Carbs-0.6 grams

Get your grapefruit on

You need 5 minutes for this

You will get one serving out of this

It's important to note here that grapefruit is only allowed on the keto diet in small doses.

What you need:

- ¼ of a grapefruit (use segments)
- ½ of a cup of cottage cheese

What you need to do to:

1. Get a bowl.
2. Place the cottage cheese at the bottom.
3. Place the grapefruit on the top.

Nutritional information:

- Calories-136
- Protein-12.5 grams
- Carbs-11.6 grams
- Fat-5.1 grams
- fiber- 1 grams

Veggie sandwich

You will need 5 minutes for this

You will get one serving

What you need:

- A single red pepper
- 2 slices of deli ham

If you need more fat in your snack, then you can add some avocado for the needed nutrition. Just note that it will change your nutritional information below.

You can also add more vegetables if you want to as well.

What you need to do:

Cut your pepper in half and take the seeds out. Place one half on a plate then stick the meat inside. Place the other half of the pepper over the top.

Nutritional information:

- Calories-101
- Protein011.2 grams
- Carbs-9.2 grams
- Fiber-2.5 grams
- Fat-2.9 grams

Cheese plate

You need five minutes for this

You will get one serving from this

What you need:

- ½ of a cup of cherry tomatoes
- An ounce of brie (this is a great cheese to use because it has no carbs)

What you need to do:

1. Place your tomatoes and cheese on a plate. If you like, you can get creative with how you do this. It looks pretty if you place the tomatoes in flower.

Nutritional information:

- Calories-133
- Fat-11.2 grams
- Carbs-2.9 grams
- Protein-4.7 grams
- Fiber-0.9 grams

Mini salad

You will need 10 minutes for this

You will get one serving from this

What you need:

- One egg (large and hard-boiled)
- ½ of a teaspoon of mustard
- A single tablespoon of mayo

What you need to do:

1. Peel the egg.
2. Mash it up well in a bowl.
3. Combine the mayo and mustard with the mashed egg.

Nutritional information

- Calorie-175
- Carbs-0.5 grams
- Protein-6.5 grams
- Fat-15 grams

Pickle wrap

You will need ten minutes for this recipe

You will get a single serving

What you need:

- A dill pill (use a large one)
- One ounce of sliced cheese
- One ounce of deli meat (sliced)

Depending on what you choose this will alter the numbers

What you need to do:

1. This is where you can get creative. You can either wrap the entire pickle with the meat and cheese, or you can cut it into slices or halves and wrap it. However, you want it to work for you.

Nutritional information:

- Calories-260
- Carbs-3 grams
- Fiber-1.5 grams
- Protein-6 grams
- Fat-9.5 grams

Meatless wraps

You will need 5 minutes for this recipe

You will get one serving from this

What you will need:

- A large collard green leaf (make sure it has no stem)
- An ounce of cheddar cheese (it will need to be sliced)
- A teaspoon of mustard (use dijon)
- A teaspoon of mayo

What you need to do:

1. Take the green leaf and spread the condiments on it before adding the cheese.
2. Then roll it like a wrap.

Nutritional information:

- Calories-162
- Fat-13.4 grams
- Carbs-1.3 grams
- Fiber-1.5 grams
- Protein-8.2 grams

Lettuce cup

You will need five minutes for this

You will get one serving

What you need to have:

- 2 ounces of tuna (canned)
- 2 tablespoons of mayo
- A lettuce leaf

What you need to do:

1. Lay the lettuce leaf flat.
2. Spread the mayo on the leaf.
3. Spread the tuna over the top.
4. Fold the lettuce into a cup shape.

Nutritional information:

- Calories-261
- Fat-22.3 grams
- Protein-13.6 grams
- Carbs-0.1 grams

Let's get Cheesy!

You will need 5 minutes for this

You will get one serving from this

What you will need:

- A quarter of a cup of cheese (use shredded and cheddar)
- 2 tablespoons of sunflower seeds
- A single can of tuna
- 2 tablespoons of mayo

What you need to do:

1. Grab a bowl.
2. Mix everything but the cheese together.
3. Add in your cheese and either leave it on the top or mix it in well as well to combine it.

Nutritional information:

- Calories-265
- Fat-21 grams
- Fiber-1 gram
- Carbs-2 grams
- Protein-17 grams

Cocoa Balls

You will need 5 minutes to make this recipe with additional time for cooling

You will get one serving from this

What you need:

- A single tablespoon of peanut butter (make sure it's natural and smooth)
- A sprinkle of cocoa powder (make sure it's unsweetened)

What you need to do:

1. Roll your peanut butter in your hands to form a ball.
2. When you have the right feel, sprinkle the ball with the powder
3. Place in a bowl and let it chill for an hour in the fridge.

Nutritional information:

- Calories-101
- Fat-8.3 grams
- Fiber-2.5 grams
- Protein-4.5 grams
- Carbs-5 grams

Veggie Sushi

You will need 20 minutes for this recipe

You will get 4 servings from this

What you need:

- 2 carrots (you need small ones, and they need to be sliced thinly)
- A quarter of an avocado (sliced thinly)
- 2 cucumbers (use medium ones and halve them)
- ½ of a bell pepper (yellow and thinly sliced)
- ½ of a bell pepper (red and thinly sliced)

If you choose to dip them, what you will need for the dip is as follows:

- A single teaspoon of soy sauce
- A single tablespoon of sriracha (for a kick in flavor)
- ⅓ of a cup of mayo

What you will need to do:

1. Use a spoon to remove the center of the cucumbers. You want them hollow.
2. Put your avocado in the center and then slide your other veggies inside that hole so that the hole is full of veggies.

3. In a small dish, make the sauce to dip the sushi in.
4. Slice the cucumber into pieces and place on a plate with the sauce.

Nutritional information:

- Calories-190
- Protein- 1 gram
- Carbs-9 grams
- Fiber-3 grams
- Fat-16 grams

Cheese bites

You will need about 20 minutes for this

You will get 4 servings for this

What you will need:

- 8 ounces of cheddar cheese (make sure that it's shredded)
- ½ teaspoon of paprika (powder)

What you will need to do:

1. Preheat your oven to 400 degrees
2. Add your cheese into a small little heaps on your baking sheet after lining it with parchment paper.
3. Make sure to leave room between each heap and that they are not touching.
4. Sprinkle your paprika over the heaps.
5. Bake for a minimum of eight minutes and a maximum of ten minutes.
6. Pay close attention that you don't burn the cheese.
7. Let them cool before you eat them.

Nutritional information:

- Calories-231
- Protein-13 grams
- Carbs-3 grams
- Fat-19 grams

Lettuce for your thoughts?

You will need five minutes for this

You will get a single serving out of this

What you will need:

- A single cherry tomato
- ½ of an ounce of butter
- A single ounce of cheese of your liking. For this recipe, we are using edam.
- 2 ounces of romaine lettuce
- ½ of an avocado

What you will need to do:

1. Make sure that you clean the lettuce thoroughly and then use the lettuce as a boat to hold the rest of the ingredients.
2. Spread butter over the lettuce, and then slice your ingredients before placing them on the top.

A fun idea is that you can put just about any vegetable or even tuna on top of the lettuce, and you will have a nutritious meal.

Nutritional information:

- Calories-374
- Protein-10 grams
- Fat-34 grams
- Carbs- 4 grams
- Fiber-8 grams

Chocolate cake

You will only need minutes for this

You will get one serving of cake from this

What you need:

- A single tablespoon of chocolate chips (use sugar-free ones)
- 2 tablespoons of melted butter
- A single tablespoon of coconut flour
- A single tablespoon of cocoa powder
- An egg that has been beaten
- ⅛ of a teaspoon of vanilla extract
- ½ a teaspoon of baking powder
- 2 tablespoons of erythritol (swerve is what we're using here)
- 2 tablespoons of almond flour
- A single pinch of salt

What you need to do:

1. Get yourself a large coffee mug.
2. Add the egg, vanilla, and egg.
3. Mix it well.
4. Add in your dry ingredients and mix it well as you did the wet ingredients.
5. Microwave on high for a minute.
6.

If you overcook it, your cake will be dry, and it won't taste right.

Nutritional information:

- Calories-397
- Fat-37 grams
- Fiber-6 grams
- Protein-12 grams

Carbs-10 grams

Conclusion

The ketogenic diet is one that has many important aspects and information that you need to know as someone who wants to try this diet. It is important to remember the warning that we have given you at the beginning of the book that this is not a diet that is safe and that doctors recommend you don't try it, or if you are going to attempt it remember that you shouldn't do so for longer than six months and even then never without the constant supervision of a doctor or at the very least a doctor knowing that your doing this and you following their guidelines and words exactly so that they can make sure that you are safe.

The ketogenic diet is a diet that believes that by minimizing your carbs, you will while maximizing the good fat in your system and making sure that you're getting the protein you need, that you will be happier and healthier. In this book we give you the information to know what this diet is all about as well as describing the different types and areas that this diet will offer. Most people assume that there is only one way to do this and while there is one thing that the additional options share, there are actually four different options you can choose from. Each one has it's unique benefits, and you should know about each type to learn what would be best for your body, which is why we have described them in the book for you to have the best information possible when you begin this diet for yourself.

Another big thing about this diet is that many people don't understand the importance of exercise with this diet. The best way to become healthier is to do three things for yourself. Get the right amount of sleep, eat healthily, and make sure that you get the proper amount of exercise as well for your body to work at an optimum level. As such we explain the exercises that are the best to go with your diet to make sure that you are getting the most out of it.

For women who are on the go and have a busy lifestyle, we have provided recipes for a thirty-day meal plan so that you can make food quickly and have a great meal for your lifestyle. They also have enough servings for you to have leftovers so that you don't have to worry about preparing in the morning. Instead, you can simply pack it up and take it with you wherever you go. This works out so much easier for so many people because they don't have to cook in the morning, and it saves a busy person a lot of time.

We also provide helpful ideas on how you can use these recipes for meals to make sure that you see how the numbers will affect you and make an impact on your day. A great example that we have explained is if you have a big breakfast that is full of the protein you need, for example, thirty grams, you've got to take note of this and be aware because if you eat too much for your dinner or another meal, you will throw your numbers out of where they are supposed to be. For those that have more time on their hands, we offer a thirty-day meal plan for you as well with all-new recipes to enjoy and tips and tricks for making them work for you in the best way.

With all of this information at your fingertips, you will be able to enjoy this diet and use it to your advantage. Another benefit that we offer? We explain routines that you can do for yourself to make this diet last longer for you and to benefit your body better as a result. Routines are very important and can be a big help to your body but also your spirit and your mind. This will help you utilize the diet better, and you will be able to improve with it as well as have it become easier for you to handle.

As many people are using this diet to their benefit, knowing your food is one of the biggest parts of this, and it becomes easier once you begin to use this in your daily life. One of the best things you can do is pay attention to the food that your eating and how it affects your body and mind. You will notice that this diet has the ability to make you sick, which isn't a good thing and it's one of the things the doctors warn against. For this reason it's very important to pay attention to what your eating and how your feeling at the same time. Another warning that we have said you need to pay attention to is that you will need to make sure that your ketogenic 'flu' isn't the result of something more serious. As people are being told that this is normal, this book has brought you the knowledge you need to be able to tell you why it's not.

This book has given you all the information you need to do this diet properly and to do it well. It's important to understand what you're getting into when you go into this diet, and this book will give you valuable information that you can use to your benefit and so you can avoid the problems that can come with this diet. You want to stay healthy and make sure that your body is able to do what it needs to. As with anything, we have put a strong emphasis on the fact that if anything feels wrong or unnatural you will need to see a doctor to make sure that you are safe and that your body can handle this diet. Use the knowledge in this book to have amazing recipes and learn how to prepare amazing meals for yourself.

Intermittent Fasting for Women

The Complete Guide to Mastering Healthy Weight Loss Using Fasting to Promote Longevity, Detox Your Body & Increase Your Energy by Way of Autophagy.

by

Dorothy Smith PhD

Introduction

Welcome to Intermittent Fasting for Women! The book where you will learn all of the information you need to begin changing your life by harnessing the concepts of autophagy and fasting.

With so many diets all over the internet and being discussed in different circles, it can be very confusing and overwhelming to know what will work for you and what won't, what research you can trust and cannot trust and where to begin once you have decided to begin. In this book, We will begin by looking at the science of intermittent fasting so that you can feel confident that you understand exactly what intermittent fasting does to your body. As well as how exactly it works to change your body composition and improve your health. This book will not push you in any certain direction, but will instead lay out all of the facts for you based on relevant studies and research, and it will leave you with this information on which you can base your decision about what kind of diet you will or will not follow, and what type of intermittent fasting regime you will choose if you decide that intermittent fasting is right for you.

We will begin by defining intermittent fasting and how it works, and then we will examine the biological methods by which it works. After you understand these concepts in detail, we will look at some specific methods that people commonly choose to follow while intermittent fasting. We will then look at the numerous benefits that intermittent fasting can provide you with including reducing your risk of disease, aiding weight loss, reducing inflammation, improving your hormone levels, and other benefits that will positively impact women over the age of 40 in particular. I will share with you some pros and cons of intermittent fasting and some tips and tricks for ensuring success if you decide that intermittent fasting is right for you. As a woman over the age of 40, you may be concerned that intermittent fasting research has not been optimized for your age and your sex. In this book, I have brought together the best in intermittent fasting research all in one place for you to review and examine so that you do not have to worry if this was optimized for you or not-because you can be confident that this book was written with you in mind!

What you put in your body and when you put it in is very important, as you will learn over the course of the next eleven chapters. This is why you must make informed choices about everything you are going to ingest, including drinks, food, snacks, supplements and pills of any sort. It can be overwhelming with the wealth of information out there to know what to listen to and what not to. This book compiles everything in one place so that you don't have to sift through pages and pages of different websites online or pages and pages of books mentioning conflicting theories regarding intermittent fasting for women. In this book, all of the information is selected and researched with health in mind as the number one priority.

Chapter 1: Intermittent Fasting

Fasting is the practice of restricting one's intake of food for a period of time, usually less than 24 hours. You may have heard of the term fasting before, as it is often associated with religious holidays and practices or fad diets you hear about in the media. The reasons why people choose to fast are widely varied, and in this book, we are going to talk about fasting in an effort to improve one's health, reduce the risk of disease and achieve or maintain a healthy body weight. The reason why people would choose to fast in order to improve their health is related to autophagy, which you are quite familiar with at this point. Fasting and autophagy go hand in hand.

The most common way to induce autophagy in a person is by way of starvation. This is not to say that a person must starve themselves, but that they starve their cells of nutrition temporarily. This is why people turn to fasting in order to induce autophagy. Low nutrition levels within the cells are the most common way that autophagy is triggered, as it is a process that creates energy within the cell. By knowing this, scientists have concluded that by inducing starvation within the cells, one can intentionally upregulate autophagy in their body.

What is Intermittent Fasting?

Intermittent Fasting (IF) is the practice of fasting for periods of time, then eating for periods of time and cycling through this repeatedly. As the name states, you are fasting intermittently. These periods of fasting and eating can vary, but are usually somewhere around twelve hours of each, cycled every day. Other examples of intermittent fasting regimes could be fasting for 16 hours in a day and then an eating window of 8 hours. In general, when you practice IF, you will separate your day or your week into eating and fasting sections of time, which will repeat either every day or every week. With this type of fasting, you are able to ingest liquids that have zero calories like water, coffee tea and any others with no caloric content. Just be sure that you drink your coffee or tea black as adding sugar will null your fast.

Myths Related to Fasting

As intermittent fasting is a relatively new area of research, this comes with many myths that must be debunked before we can go further into our discussion of the topic. Before moving onto the chapters that follow in the remainder of this book, we will look at some common myths concerning fasting.

Myth 1: Fasting Lets You Eat Whatever You Want

A common myth around fasting is that because you are fasting, you are able to eat whatever you want when you finally do begin eating again. This mindset can lead people to eat things like fast food or high amounts of sugar when they break their fast. These high calorie foods that the person thinks they are now able to eat due to having fasted can lead to them not achieving their goals and even in some cases to gain weight.

Myth 2: Fasting Lets You Eat As Much As You Want

Another myth, similar to the first one and which goes hand in hand with it, is the belief that fasting allows a person to then eat in whatever quantity they want when they break their fast. This can cause people to grossly overeat because they will tend to eat in larger quantities after a fast as they are quite hungry and because their brain tells them to eat more in order to prepare for a possible subsequent fast.

Myth 3: Fasting Will Give Everyone The Same Results

When it comes to health and techniques involving the body, there is no technique that will work for everyone in the exact same way. When it comes to the body, everyone's will react differently and will show different changes on its own timeline. When you are trying something new in an effort to elicit changes from your body, you must keep in mind that your body is unique and individual.

There are many different ways to fast and different ideas of what are the most effective ways. Trying things with a flexible mindset will help you to find the way that works best for you.

Myth 4: Your Body Only Digests at Certain Times of the Day

There is a common misconception about why fasting works. This misconception is that your body can only digest food at certain times of the day and that fasting works around these times. This is not true, however. Many people believe that digestion does not occur during the night, but in reality, digestion will occur no matter what time of day you ingest food. The purpose of fasting is to allow your body enough time for digestion as well as other processes before you eat again. We will look at this in more depth in the next chapter. It is important to keep in mind though that the body does not take breaks from completing its processes, and by changing the times that you ingest food, you are working with these ongoing processes to try to achieve a desired outcome.

Myth 5: Fasting Will Break Down Your Muscles

While your body will sometimes begin breaking down parts like fat for energy, this does not happen the same way with muscle. Fat is stored to be used for fuel for the body later on, and when we are fasting, this is often what occurs. When we are eating regularly throughout the day, the body will use the sugars you are eating for fuel. It is very rare that your body does not have enough sugar or enough fat stores to use as energy. Therefore it is very rare that the body will begin using muscle for energy. Muscle takes a long time to break down for energy, and it is very necessary for the body to have muscle, so this myth is something that you should not fear when considering fasting.

Myth 6: Fasting Will Leave You Malnourished

Fasting for a short period of time with an end in sight (like 12 hours or 16 hours) will not lead you to lose your nutrients and vitamin stores that your body needs. Keep in mind, our bodies are very smart machines designed for survival, and they will not easily let go of things that are beneficial to its survival. Further, when you do break your fast, you will replenish your body's nutrients and minerals that it did not get during your fast. There is no need to worry about becoming malnourished due to fasting as long as you are eating a healthy and balanced diet when you eventually break your fast.

Now that we have debunked several myths about fasting, we will begin to look into several topics related to fasting in more detail. The first step (which we will visit in the next chapter) is knowing what autophagy is and how it functions, before learning how you can take advantage of this natural process to improve your health.

Chapter 2: Autophagy

In this chapter, we will look at something that is likely a new topic for you. This topic is called Autophagy. We are going to examine autophagy as it plays a crucial role in intermittent fasting and understanding the science behind why intermittent fasting works will help you to feel confident and comfortable as you change your diet and lifestyle to accommodate this new regime.

What is Autophagy

Autophagy itself is a process that happens within the body, and that has been going on since the beginning of humans. It is only recently that people began harnessing this process to achieve desired positive results. We will look at this topic in-depth throughout this book but here we will begin by looking at what exactly Autophagy is.

Autophagy, as a word, can be broken up into two individual parts. Each of these parts on its own is a separate Greek word. The word auto, which means *self* and the word phagy which means *the practice of eating.* Putting these together gives you *the practice of self-eating,* which is essentially what autophagy is. Now this may sound like some type of new-age cannibalism, but it is a very natural process that our cells practice all the time without us being any the wiser. Autophagy is the body's way of cleaning itself out.

The process of autophagy involves small "hunter" particles that go around your body, looking for cells or cell components that are old and damaged. The hunter particles then take these cell components apart, getting rid of the damaged parts and saving the useful parts to make new cells later. These hunter cells can also use the leftover useful parts to create energy for the body.

Autophagy has been found to happen in all organisms that are multi-cellular, like animals and plants, in addition to humans. While the study of these larger organisms and how autophagy works in their cells is lesser-known, more studies are being done on humans and how changes in diet can affect their body's autophagy.

The other function that autophagy serves is that it helps cells to carry out their death when it is time for them to die. There are times when cells are programmed to die, because of a number of different factors. Sometimes these cells need assistance in their death, and autophagy can help them with this or can help to clean up after their death. The human body is all about life and death and these processes are continually going on without our knowledge to keep us healthy and in good form.

As I mentioned, the process of autophagy has been going on inside of us for many, many years, since the beginning of humans. This process has been kept around inside of our bodies because of the multitude of benefits it can provide us with. It is also essential for the health of our bodies, as being able to get rid of waste and damaged parts that are no longer useful to us is essential to our health. If we were unable to get rid of damaged or broken cells, these damaged particles would build up and eventually make us sick. Our bodies are extremely efficient in everything that they do, and waste disposal is no different.

It is in more recent years that the study of autophagy has been focused more heavily on in terms of diet and disease research. These studies are still in their early stages as it has been only a few years shy of sixty years since autophagy was discovered. This process was discovered in a lab by testing what happened when small organisms went without food for some time. These organisms were observed very closely under a microscope, and it was found that their cells had this process of waste disposal and energy creation that was later named autophagy.

More about autophagy and its relation to energy production is being studied in recent years, as this topic is of interest to humans. Autophagy can use old cell parts and recycle them to create new energy that the organism (like the human or animal) can then use to do its regular functions like walking and breathing. Now, people are studying what happens when humans rely on this form of energy production instead of the energy they would get from ingesting food throughout the day. This is where autophagy and Intermittent fasting come together. We will look at how they work together throughout the rest of this book as we delve deeply into intermittent fasting and autophagy and how they work together to allow for things like weight loss or disease prevention.

What is the Function of Autophagy?

Autophagy has many functions in the body. In the previous section on "what is autophagy," you learned that it is a process that helps to discard old and damaged cells and use their parts for energy. In this section, we will look at some of the other functions of autophagy and the body systems involved.

Autophagy is said to be the housekeeping function of the body. If you think of your body as your home, autophagy is the housekeeper that you hire to take care of all of the waste and the recycling functions of your cells.

One of the housekeeping duties includes removing cell parts that were built wrongly or at the wrong time. Sometimes cells make mistakes, and these mistakes can cause proteins or other cell parts to be formed in error. When this happens, we need something within the cell to get rid of these so that they do not take up space or get in the way of other processes within the cell. Further, sometimes useful parts of the cell will become damaged somehow and then will need to be removed in order to make way for a new part to take its place. These cell parts can include those that create DNA or those that create the proteins needed to make the DNA.

Another duty of autophagy is to protect the body from disease and pathogens. Pathogens are bacteria or viruses that can infect our cells and our bodies if they are not properly defended against. Autophagy works to kill the cells within our body that are infected by these pathogens in order to get rid of them before they can spread. In this way, autophagy plays a part in our immune system as it acts as a supplement to our immune cells whose sole function is to protect us from invasions by disease and infection.

Autophagy also functions to help the cells of the body to regulate themselves when there are stressors placed upon them. These stressors can be things like a lack of food for the cell or physical stresses placed on the cell. This regulation helps to maintain a standard cell environment despite factors that can change, like the availability of food. Autophagy is able to do things like break down cell parts for food to provide the cell with nutrients.

Similar to its role in regulation of the cells, autophagy also helps with the development of a growing fetus inside of a woman's uterus. Autophagy occurs here to ensure that the embryo has enough nutrients and energy at all times for healthy development. In addition to this, it helps with growth in adults as well as there is a balance of building new parts and breaking down old ones involved in the growth of any organism.

Autophagy is more important than we may even realize, as it plays a large role in the survival of the living organisms it acts within. It does this by being especially sensitive to the levels of nutrients and energy within a cell. When the nutrient levels lower, autophagy breaks down cell parts which create nutrients and energy for the cell. If it weren't for this process, the cells would not be able to maintain their ideal functioning environment and they may begin to make more mistakes and even lower their functioning abilities altogether. So much goes on inside of a cell that they need to be able to work effectively at all times. Autophagy makes this possible which is what makes it such an essential function.

How Does Autophagy Work in the Body

Autophagy functions in the following way. When a decrease in nutrients is noticed within a cell, this decrease in nutrients acts as a signal for the cell to create small pockets within a membrane (a thin barrier layer) that are called *autophagosome*s. These small pockets (autophagosomes) move through the cell and find debris and damaged particles floating around within the cell. The small pockets then consume this debris by absorbing it into its inner space. The debris is then enclosed in the membrane (the thin barrier layer) and is moved to a place in the cell called the Lysosome. A lysosome is a part of a cell that acts as a center for degradation, breakdown, or disassembly. This part of the cell gets debris and damaged cell parts delivered to it by the autophagosomes. Once these damaged cell parts are delivered, the lysosomes then break them down. By breaking them down, these parts can be recycled and used for energy.

Two Types of Autophagy

There are two different forms of autophagy- Macroautophagy and Microautophagy. These two different types act in slightly different ways.

Macroautophagy

For the most part, when you hear or see the word autophagy, it is in reference to *Macroautophagy.* This is the form that is most often discussed in relation to things like diet and health.

Microautophagy

Microautophagy differs from Macroautophagy slightly in the way that it works. While both still accomplish the same end goal, the way that they get there is what sets them apart from each other. In the type of autophagy that we discussed in the previous section, small pockets surrounded by membranes called autophagosomes are created, and they take up debris in the cell and move it to the lysosomes to be broken down and used for energy. When it comes to Microautophagy, the difference is that the debris floating around within the cell moves to the lysosome on its own without being carried there inside of an autophagosome. Once it reaches the lysosome, it is engulfed by the membrane of the lysosome and then is taken inside to be broken down.

Sometimes the way that this debris reaches the lysosome in Microautophagy is not *totally* on its own, as there is a protein complex that escorts or chaperones it to the lysosome. If there is a signal of low nutrient levels within the cell and Microautophagy is needed in addition to Macroautophagy, then the chaperone proteins may search out debris within the cell and escort it to the lysosome to be taken inside. The chaperone protein will then leave to find more debris to escort back to the lysosome.

Macroautophagy Versus Microautophagy

Now that you know that there are two different types of autophagy and the difference between them, you may be wondering which one occurs when and which of these two we are more concerned with when it comes to disease and health.

Both of these processes are occurring regularly within our cells, and the frequency with which each of them occurs must create a balance. This balance must be created for one very important reason. When the small pockets called autophagosomes are created and they move to the lysosome, they attach their membrane to the membrane of the lysosome in order to drop off the debris that they contain. Then, once the debris is dropped off, this new membrane that has attached itself is left there, thus becoming a part of the membrane of the lysosome. This increases the size of the lysosome membrane by a bit of length each time. When Microautophagy occurs, the debris meets the outside of the lysosome and is taken into the lysosome by being engulfed by the membrane of the lysosome which creates a small pocket inside of the lysosome that contains the debris. This new small pocket has been created by the lysosome membrane, meaning that the lysosome membrane has become shorter in length by a small amount. Because of the way these two types of autophagy act, they must happen at about the same frequency as each other so that the size of the lysosome membrane can remain consistent. If this was not the case, we would either be left with a much larger lysosome due to increased lysosome membrane size after Macroautophagy, or a much smaller lysosome in the case of Microautophagy. These two processes not only ensure that the lysosome size remains consistent, but they ensure that the debris within the cell is broken down and recycled as efficiently as possible.

Ketosis

Ketosis is a state that the body enters when there is a lack of recently-ingested sugars (carbohydrates) or stored sugars, and it must instead use stored fat to get its energy. When the body enters this state, it breaks down its fat stores and the breakdown of these fat stores creates an acid as a by-product. This acid that is created is called a *Ketone*. When in a state of ketosis, the brain is able to use ketones for energy instead of carbohydrates or sugars like it normally would.

This state of ketosis in the brain induces autophagy in the brain cells, which has many benefits for the brain. The way that this works is that the Ketones in the brain induce autophagy by signaling to the brain cells that there are low levels of energy sources, which is why the brain is using ketones for energy. If you remember, low energy levels are a signal for autophagy. It is not completely understood much further than this. But ketosis and its induction of autophagy in the brain has produced many positive effects for the brain like the protection of brain cells. This leads to a reduction in the likelihood of diseases like Alzheimer's or Parkinson's.

What Triggers Autophagy

1. Starvation

The most common way to induce autophagy in a person is by way of starvation. Autophagy is triggered by a decrease in nutrients within a cell. As I mentioned above, this decrease in nutrients acts as a signal within the cell to begin the process of autophagy.

2. Aerobic Exercise

One other way to activate autophagy is through exercise. Aerobic exercise has been shown through studies to increase autophagy in the cells of the muscles, the heart, the brain, lungs, and the liver.

3. Sleep

Sleep is very important for autophagy. If you have ever gone a few days without proper, restful sleep, you know that you begin to feel a decline in your mental abilities rather quickly. This could be because of your brain's decreased autophagy functioning. The number of hours that you are in bed does not matter if the sleep is not good quality though. Quality sleep for the right number of hours is what is needed to maintain good brain function and keep your brain's autophagy going.

4. Specific Foods

The consumption of specific foods has been shown to induce or promote autophagy. We will look at some examples of these foods below. The added benefit is that not only do they trigger autophagy in the cells of your body, these foods are also shown to have numerous other health benefits.

- **Coffee**

It may come as a surprise, but coffee and caffeine, in general, have been shown to induce autophagy, specifically within the brain. It is not only the caffeine that promotes autophagy; however, as decaffeinated coffee has also proven to induce autophagy in the brain. The antioxidants in coffee are one component of it that promotes autophagy, along with the caffeine. The combination of coffee and the caffeine it contains make regular caffeinated coffee a great food to trigger autophagy in the brain. The caffeine in coffee induces autophagy in the brain which acts to protect against disorders of the brain such as Alzheimer's or dementia.

- **The Coffee Cherry**

Similarly to the example of coffee above, the actual coffee cherry from which the coffee beans are extracted is also loaded with beneficial components that are great for promoting autophagy in the brain. In addition to the beans themselves and the caffeine and antioxidants they contain, the actual cherry fruit contains many other elements that are beneficial to the brain and brain health.

- **Green Tea**

Green tea is another beverage that has been found to induce autophagy in the brain. Green tea contains some caffeine, which you now know induces autophagy, thus protecting the brain, but it also contains another antioxidant which is different from that found in coffee. This antioxidant is called EGCG and is known for its positive effects on the brain. EGCG triggers autophagy in brain cells which also cleans the brain of degeneration and clears toxic cells which prevent disorders of the brain and keeps the brain functioning as well as possible. The way that green tea triggers autophagy is also beneficial for memory and learning. The benefits of green tea are far-reaching because of and in addition to its effect on autophagy.

- **Coconut Oil**

Coconut oil is another extremely beneficial food to ingest in order to improve and maintain a healthy brain through autophagy. Coconut oil is beneficial as it increases the number of ketones in the brain, which, as you learned in the previous chapter, is beneficial for autophagy because ketones in the brain induce autophagy by signaling to the brain cells that there are low levels of energy sources.

Coconut oil can be ingested in a number of ways which is what makes it such a great food for the brain. You can use coconut oil as cooking oil, in place of a cooking spray, as a substitute in baking, in your coffee, in smoothies and on your skin.

- **Ginger**

Ginger is known to be healthy for humans for a number of reasons, such as its amazing ability to treat nausea, its pain relieving properties and its benefits for reducing inflammation. In addition to this, it contains a compound called 6-shogaol which has numerous benefits itself including its ability to induce autophagy. 6-shogaol also has been shown to reduce the risk of developing cancer as it is an anti-tumor agent as it is able to prevent the uncontrolled growth of cells that develops into a tumor. This is not studied to its full capacity yet, but this ability to stop tumor growth could be due to its effects on autophagy.

Ginger can be ingested in a variety of ways as well, such as in a powder form, as a plant in tea or in cooking both savory and sweet foods. Many Asian dishes incorporate ginger because of its numerous health benefits.

- **Galangal**

Galangal is very similar to ginger in the way that it looks, which is why it is often referred to as "thai ginger," however it is actually different than ginger in the way that it tastes. Galangal is not the same as ginger in its wide range of health benefits, but it is similar in that is contains an active compound that induces autophagy in the brain. Further, it is able to specifically benefit the cells associated with dopamine, which is a hormone that leads us to feel happy. This means that Galangal could prove to have benefits for treating depression as well, due to its ability to protect these dopamine-associated brain cells through its induction of autophagy.

- **Reishi Mushroom**

The Reishi Mushroom is a specific type of mushroom that, like ginger, has many bioactive components. Bioactive means that it has compounds within it that have an effect on biological organisms like humans. When ingested, these bioactive compounds exert their effects on the body, such as inducing autophagy for example. This Reishi mushroom, in particular, is able to induce autophagy as well as to regulate it. This means that it is able to cause autophagy to occur as well as regulating the amount and duration of it.

The Reishi mushroom is no new discovery, as it has been used in Chinese medicine for thousands of years as a way of improving immune system function, reducing inflammation, and improving the functioning of the brain. All of these areas that the Reishi mushroom has been known to help are also areas that are impacted by autophagy, which can give us insight into the mechanism by which the bioactive compounds in this mushroom operate.

The Reishi mushroom can be used in cooking or taken in a tincture form for a concentrated dose of the bioactive compounds.

- **Turmeric**

Turmeric is a rather popular spice in the western world today, found in all types of drinks and foods. This is no new discovery either, though, as it is found in Indian curries and has been for decades. Turmeric is so powerful as a spice because it is able to induce autophagy in the brain which protects them from damage as it clears out damaged cells in order for new ones to replace them.

Turmeric can be found in food like curry, in baking, and in many different sorts of drinks such as tea or in turmeric lattes in virtually every coffee shop these days. Turmeric has a very strong yellow-orange hue that is unmistakable.

- **Brussels Sprouts, Cabbage, Kale, Broccoli Sprouts**

All of these green vegetables have one thing in common- they all contain Sulforaphane. Sulforaphane is a plant chemical that is found naturally in these vegetables. This is an antioxidant that acts in a similar way to turmeric and thus has similar benefits. Sulforaphane like turmeric, induces autophagy in the brain which helps to reduce the risk of Alzheimer's, Parkinson's and dementia which are all neurodegenerative diseases. *Neurodegenerative* means that the cells in the brain called nerves are damaged and broken down, which leads to cognitive decline like Alzheimer's or physical decline as in Parkinson's. These vegetables can help to treat these diseases by slowing their progression, as they are all diseases that come about over time. There is no cure yet, but the treatment at this stage involves delaying the progression of these diseases.

Sulforaphane can be found in the aforementioned vegetables, but the strongest source is in broccoli sprouts. It can also be taken concentrated in a supplement form.

- **Extra Virgin Olive Oil**

Olive oil and extra virgin olive oil, in particular, is beneficial to the health of humans because it has positive effects on inflammation. It is able to reduce inflammation in the brain and the body as well as improve brain functioning as it is able to induce autophagy in the brain. Because of this, extra virgin olive oil, like Sulforaphane is recommended as a treatment to slow the progression of Alzheimer's disease.

Olive oil can be used for cooking, as a dressing, as a dip and even ingested on its own as a dietary supplement.

- **Acai Berries, Strawberries and Blueberries**

The bioactive compounds in these specific types of berries work in the brain to induce autophagy and reduce inflammation. This leads to the protection of brain cells in this case from *oxidative stress*. Oxidative stress is something that can happen within the brain when there is an imbalance of oxygen, which can cause reduced cognitive functioning. These berries and their induction of autophagy helps to reduce this by keeping the balance of oxygen at a healthy level.

- **Omega-3 Fatty Acids**

Omega-3 Fatty Acids are fats that are needed in your diet as the body cannot make them on its own. These fatty acids are a certain type in a list of other fatty acids, but this type (Omega-3) are the most essential and the most beneficial for our brains. They have numerous effects on the brain, including reducing inflammation (which reduces the risk of

Alzheimer's) and maintaining and improving mood and cognitive function, including memory. Omega-3's have these greatly beneficial effects because of the way that they act in the brain, which is what makes them so essential to our diets.

Omega-3 Fatty Acids increase the production of new nerve cells in the brain by acting specifically on the nerve stem cells within the brain, causing new and healthy nerve cells to be generated. It does this by a combination of actions, including inducing autophagy in the brain.

Omega-3 fatty acids can be found in fish like salmon, sardines, black cod, and herring. It can also be taken as a pill-form supplement for those who do not eat fish or cannot eat enough of it. It can also be taken in the form of a fish oil supplement like krill oil.

Omega-3's are by far the most important dietary source for inducing autophagy simply because of the numerous benefits that come from it, both in the brain and in the rest of the body. While supplements are often a last step when it comes to trying to include something in your diet, for Omega-3's, the benefits are too great to potentially miss by trying to receive all of it from your diet.

As you can see, there are many different ways to optimize autophagy. The way or ways that you choose will be highly dependent on you as an individual. You may want to approach this by trying one and being open to changing methods if it does not work as well as you would like. You may want to try a combination of methods in order to get the best results. The key is to be flexible and be open to change, as nobody knows how their body will react to changes in diet and exercise.

The reason why it is important for you to learn these details about the functioning of autophagy and the different types that occur and when is because by knowing how these things work within your body, you are able to understand how changing specific things like when you eat and when you fast will impact the functioning of your cells. By blindly following someone's advice about what you should do with your own body, especially something like when to practice fasting, you will not be able to properly understand the results you see or the reasons why you may not see results. You may then become frustrated that the advice you took isn't working. However, the best way to approach something like this is to learn everything you can about your body and how it works before making changes. Then, once you have understood this, begin to make changes that you understand. By doing this, when you begin to see changes, whether positive or negative, you can make small adjustments to your plan and monitor your progress. If we take advice without understanding why we are doing it, we may be left feeling discouraged and confused.

Chapter 3: Types of Intermittent Fasting

Now that you know what autophagy is and how it works, as well as how it can malfunction and create disease, we are going to look at how you can harness it and manipulate it in order to improve your health and reduce your chance of disease.

In order to harness and manipulate autophagy to benefit your body, you need to be able to upregulate its functioning within your cells. There are various ways to do this, and we will look at these ways in this chapter, as well as how they work so that you can better understand how they work to affect your body. By upregulating autophagy, you are able to make your body resistant to many diseases, as you will learn later on in this book.

Water Fasting

The first type of fasting we will look at is water fasting. Water fasting is a method of fasting in which a person does not ingest anything except water for a period of time. Many people practice water fasting for periods up to 72 hours, but this is a decision that should be made with the help of a doctor.

If you have ever gone into the hospital for a medical procedure, they likely told you that you could not eat food and could only drink water for a certain amount of time before the procedure. This practice would have been a form of water fasting. Some people also try water fasting as a method of "detoxing" their bodies. Another use for it though is to manually induce autophagy. Many people practice periods of water fasting to induce autophagy in order to rid their body of potentially harmful viruses or bacteria in an effort to reduce their risk of diseases such as cancer and Alzheimer's and even increase their lifespan. This is because of the cleansing properties of autophagy, as it breaks down infected cells and uses their salvageable parts for new and healthy cells to be generated. As you know from reading the previous chapter, autophagy can have a profound effect on cancer. Autophagy can reduce the risk of cancers because of the way that it clears the body of damaged cells, which could otherwise accumulate and develop into cancer.

There are added benefits of water fasting that do not directly involve autophagy, but that is worth noting anyway. Water fasting has been shown to reduce blood pressure, cholesterol and even improve the functioning of insulin in the body, therefore improving blood sugar.

The problem with water fasting is that it can be quite dangerous if not practiced in a safe and monitored way. Consult a doctor before attempting a water fast so that you can ensure you are doing so in a safe way. There are some groups of people who should not practice water fasting. These groups include pregnant women, children, the elderly, and people with eating disorders.

Another thing to keep in mind when attempting a water fast in an effort to lose weight is that the weight lost during a water fast may not be the exact type of weight that you are trying to lose. During a water fast, there is a severe restriction in calories, which leads to the breakdown of fat stores, but some of the weight loss could also include water weight, stored carbohydrates and sometimes muscle (in longer fasts). What this means is that after a water fast, the weight loss may come back quite quickly if the majority was water or carbohydrate stores, as these are replenished very quickly once a person begins eating again. If this is the case, do not be concerned, this is a very normal reaction for your body to have as it is built to anticipate unexpected fasts and therefore has ways to protect you from these, such as storing carbohydrates.

When approaching a water fast, it is beneficial to prepare your body for a few days leading up to it by tapering off your eating portions in order to gradually remove food from your day. This will better prepare your body to go without food for a day or two. Another way to get your body prepared to water fast is to fast for part of the day so that it can get accustomed to spending some time without food. You may also be wondering how a water fast could make you lose water weight, but it is entirely possible and even likely. This is because much of the water we bring into our bodies throughout the day is enclosed in the foods we eat. If your water intake remains the same, but your food ingestion dramatically decreases, you could end up becoming dehydrated and thus losing water weight.

You will also need to adjust your activities to accommodate this water fast, especially if it is your first time trying it. If you are not used to fasting, you may feel dizzy or light-headed, and this may make some of your daily tasks more difficult. This could be due to lower blood sugar or lower blood pressure if you are dehydrated. Be sure to keep this in mind as you attempt a water fast and be sure to increase your water intake to avoid a drop in blood pressure.

There is still much more research that needs to be done surrounding water fasting in humans in particular. Water fasting as a method of weight loss is a relatively new approach and one that is just beginning to be explored with human test subjects.

16 And 8

This is the method I briefly mentioned where you would eat for 8 hours of the day and fast for 16 hours. When doing this method of IF, you would usually skip breakfast and eat between the hours of 1pm and 9pm, or 12 noon and 8pm. The hours you choose can vary depending on your work schedule and your lifestyle, but the key is that you eat for 8 hours of the day and have a longer portion of the day in which you are fasting. This is the most popular method of IF and is the easiest if you are new to following specific diets. Many people will naturally eat during an 8-hour window of the day if they do not tend to eat breakfast, which is why this method is the easiest to transition to. Some people prefer to use different ranges of hours, but in terms of research, 16 and 8 has been shown to be the most effective. If you are looking for something a little different, we will look at the two next most common methods below.

5:2

This method is different from the other two in that it involves a number of calories instead of hours. However, similar to the previous method, you are breaking up your week into different days instead of breaking up your day into hours.

In this method, you will restrict your caloric intake to between 500 and 600 calories on two days of the week. This is similar to the Eat-Stop-Eat method, except that instead of fully fasting on Monday and Thursday (for example), you will greatly restrict your caloric intake. For the other five days of the week, you will eat as you normally would. This is a method of intermittent eating, though it does not involve complete fasting. This method would be good for those who are unable to completely fast for two days of the week but who want to try a form of intermittent eating still. For example, this would be a good option for someone who works a physically laborious job and who cannot be feeling light-headed during the workday.

Eat- Stop- Eat

This method is a little different than the 16 and 8 method, as instead of breaking the day up into hours, you would be breaking your week up into days. You would fast for either one or two days of the week, not on back-to-back days. For example, you would fast from after lunch on Monday until after lunch on Tuesday and then again beginning after lunch on Thursday. For all the other days of the week, you could eat normally as you wish. This type is similar to water fasting in that it is a period of time where you are fasting, which is 24 hours in length. However, it is intermittent in that it only lasts 24 hours and repeats itself twice every week consistently. A water fast could be a one-off for 72 hours.

With this method, you will have to keep in mind that what you choose to eat and in what quantities on the days that you are not fasting will have effects on the results you see. You want to ensure you are not bingeing on the days that you are not fasting. More on this in chapter 8 though. This method is a good choice for those who prefer more flexibility during their eating times and do not want to restrict their eating to a small 8-hour window of the day, namely those who want to eat breakfast. This could be good for those who have longer working days and who prefer to have a longer time to eat during the day.

Alternate Day Fasting

This method of fasting involves fasting every other day and eating normally on the non-fasting days. Similar to other forms of IF, you are able to drink as much as you want of calorie-free drinks such as black coffee, tea, and water. You would fast for 24 hours on your fasting days, for example, from before dinner on one day until before dinner the next day. This method can be very successful or very unsuccessful depending on the person. The problem with this method is that it can lead to bingeing on the non-fasting days. If, however, you are a person that does not tend to binge, you may enjoy the flexibility that this diet offers by allowing you to eat whatever you want on alternating days.

There is a modification that some people choose to apply to this form of IF, where they allow themselves to eat 500 calories on their fasting days. This works out to about 20-25% of an adult person's daily energy needs, which will still put you in an extreme calorie deficit for those days, leading to the induction of autophagy. This method allows a person to continue with this diet consistently for a longer period of time than they may be able to with full fasts. It has the same effectiveness and works better with our modern lifestyles.

This type of IF has been shown to be very beneficial for weight loss and is a good choice for those who have weight loss as their main priority. Because of the calorie deficit that it put a person into, they are using more energy than they are putting into their body, which leads to a breakdown of fat stores and weight loss.

Women-Specific Methods of Intermittent Fasting

There is some evidence that suggests that Intermittent Fasting affects the bodies of men and women differently. The bodies of women are much more sensitive to small calorie changes, especially small negative changes in the intake of calories. Since the bodies of women are made for conceiving and growing babies, women's bodies must be sensitive to any sort of changes that may occur in the internal environment of the body to a larger degree than the bodies of men, in order to ensure that it will produce healthy and strong progeny. For this reason, however, some women may have trouble practicing intermittent fasting according to the above methods. These methods may involve too much restriction for the body of a woman, and she may feel some negative effects such as light-headedness or fatigue. In order to prevent this, there are some adjusted methods of intermittent fasting that will work better for women's bodies. This is not to say that women cannot practice IF or fasting of any sort, but that they must keep this in mind when deciding to try a fasting diet. Women can take a modified approach to fasting so that the internal environment of their bodies remains healthy. There are some slightly different patterns of IF that may be safer and more beneficial for women. We will look at these below.

Crescendo

This method is quite similar to the Eat-Stop-Eat method that we discussed earlier, except that in this one, the hours have been changed slightly. This fasting regimen involves breaking up the week into days as well as breaking up the days into hours. In this case, the woman would fast for 14 to 16 hours of the day twice a week and eating normally every other day. These fasting days would not be back to back and would not be more than twice per week.

Alternate Day 5:2

Alternatively, she could fast every other day but only for 12-14 hours, eating normally on the days in between. On the fasting days, she would eat 25% of her normal calorie intake, making it a reduction in calories and not a full-blown fast.

14 and 10

This is a modification of the 16 and 8 method described earlier. In this method, the day would be broken up into segments of hours. The woman would fast for 14 hours of the day and eat for 10 hours. Beginning with this modified version will allow her body to become used to fasting. Eventually, when she is comfortable with it, she can change the hours by one hour per day in order to reach 16 and 8.

By reducing the hours of the fast to fourteen hours or less, women can still experience the benefits that IF can have for weight loss and autophagy induction without putting themselves in any danger. This is not to say that women cannot fast in the same way that men can, but that they must start off slowly and gradually increase their hours of fasting so that they do not shock their bodies. When it comes to health, we must acknowledge the fact that the bodies of men and women are built differently and thus will respond differently to changes.

12 and 12

Women can also benefit from reducing their fasting window even further to 12 hours. This method can be beneficial in the beginning while your body gets used to the fasting, and you can gradually work your way up from here. In this method, you would normally only eat until three hours before you go to sleep, and then you could begin eating again early enough in the morning to have your first meal be breakfast. For example, if you go to bed at 10pm, you would only eat until 7pm. Then you could eat breakfast after 7am. This is beneficial for people who like to eat breakfast and who do not like to begin their day fasted.

For any person, regardless of their sex, the best approach to fasting may vary. When it comes to choosing an approach, being flexible is important. With dieting, the most important factor is consistency and so the best diet that you can choose for yourself will be the one that you can consistently maintain for a long enough period of time that your body can adjust, and changes can begin to occur.

Chapter 4: The Pros and Cons of Intermittent Fasting

For any of the populations described above, seeking medical advice before beginning any type of fasting is necessary. Your doctor will be able to examine your specific case and determine if fasting is possible for you and if you should attempt it. Remember, fasting is done to improve health (with the exception of for religious reasons), so if it is detrimental to your health, then there is likely no point in pursuing it. The bottom line is that you must take care of your health and each person is an individual. Before you try anything new involving your health, consulting a healthcare professional that knows your specific case is the best way to protect your body.

For those who are in generally good health, you still may want to consult a doctor before deciding to begin any type of fasting regimen. It may be beneficial to explore the pros and cons of a fasting diet plan with a healthcare professional so that you can make an informed decision for yourself about it. If you decide that you would like to try it, there is no harm in keeping your doctor updated every now and then so that they can monitor your health. This can also be beneficial in that they can tell you if you are making progress of any sort and give you their recommendations along the way.

Pros

We will begin by looking at the pros when it comes to intermittent fasting.

1. When you are deciding which form of fasting is best for you, it is beneficial to keep in mind that intermittent fasting can be safer than water fasting for longer periods of time (as many people do) as it involves much shorter durations of fasting, making it better for those who are not as comfortable fasting for longer periods.

2. For women, there are some benefits to fasting that are different than those for men. Most notably, are the benefits that it has on the heart for women. Things like blood pressure

and cholesterol can lead to severe and life-threatening heart diseases, and fasting has been shown to improve heart health in women.

3. It also improves the efficiency with which the bodies of women use insulin to control blood sugar.

Cons

1. There is some evidence that suggests that IF affects men and women differently. Some studies have shown that in men, IF helped their bodies to more efficiently regulate blood sugar, while in women, this was not the case and the regulation of blood sugar actually worsened. Another notable difference is that

2. Fasting, in general, may be harmful for some populations such as the elderly, women trying to conceive and people with a history of eating disorders

3. There are some populations who should not fast due to the health risks it may pose. While fasting can provide health benefits, the following groups of people should not do so without first consulting a medical professional.

- **Those who have Kidney problems**

People suffering from kidney disease need more calories than people who are in good health. They need the nutrition that these calories provide them with as well. For this reason, those with kidney problems such as kidney stones, kidney failure, or any other disease of the kidneys should not participate in fasting.

- **Those who have Liver problems**

Fasting is hard on the liver, as it is the liver that makes the ketones that the body uses for energy during fasting when carbohydrates are not available. If the liver is already stressed by disease, it is not a good idea to put further stress on the liver by then fasting.

- **Women who are trying to conceive**

When women are trying to conceive, their bodies are sensitive to the state of the internal environment of the body. This is because the body will not allow conception if the environment is not ideal for the growth of a healthy fetus. It is important to ensure that your body is in good shape and has enough nutrients if you are trying to conceive so that the body is confident in the fact that it will be able to grow a healthy baby.

- **Those who are underweight**

If you are underweight, your body will not have access to the fat stores that it would turn to in the event of a fast. In this case, fasting can be dangerous because without these fat stores to break down for energy; the body can then reach a state of severe lack of energy and nutrients

- **Those who are pregnant**

When pregnant, your body is attempting to grow a healthy baby. In order to do this, the baby cannot go without the proper nutrients and food that it needs to grow, everything that you ingest while pregnant will be shared with your baby through the umbilical cord. If you do not have enough nutrients, the development of the baby could suffer.

- **Those who are breastfeeding**

While breastfeeding, the nutrients and minerals from everything that the mother ingests are passed to the baby through the milk. There are studies that show that the taste of the breast milk can change depending on what the mother has most recently ingested. For this reason, it is important that the mother remains nourished and fed so that the baby is getting proper nourishment as well. The first few months, while the mother is breastfeeding, are essential to the development of the baby and the breast milk is the main reason for this. Keeping the breast milk full of nutrients is essential.

- **Women who have irregular periods**

It has been shown that fasting can cause women to have irregular periods due to the changes in hormone production and secretion that it can cause. Those who experience this already should avoid fasting without consulting a doctor first.

- **Those with a history of eating disorders**

For people who have a history of eating disorders of any sort, diets can be quite tricky. It is important for these people to be careful when restricting or controlling food intake in any way. Food-related planning and restricting can act as a trigger for those who have a history of eating disorders. It is not recommended that those people participate in intermittent fasting or fasting of any sort.

- **The Elderly**

The elderly are at a vulnerable age as they are more susceptible to diseases and illnesses of any sort. They also tend to be smaller in size and have less body fat than they did when they were younger. For these reasons, it is not advised that they use fasting as a form of health improvement. This population needs all of the nutrients that they receive from the foods they eat, as well as the regular blood sugar levels that come with ingesting food regularly throughout the day. As they do not have as much fat stored on their bodies, they will not have the fat to break down for energy while fasting. Because of this, fasting can be dangerous for the elderly.

- **Those who are below the age of eighteen**

For people who are in their teen years, or especially children, fasting is not a necessary tool for weight loss or health improvement. Any sort of diet that involves fasting is not advisable for this population as they are still growing and developing and are in need of all of the nutrients that they ingest. They also tend to be more active, and because of this, they likely use up more than the number of calories that they eat on a daily basis. At these ages, the body is in need of calories to allow it to grow and change in the proper ways to prepare it for adulthood.

- **Those who have conditions of the heart**

Those with conditions of the heart should take extra care if they are fasting for religious reasons, and otherwise should avoid fasting altogether.

This is because their medication schedule is very rigid, and it must be taken with food. As this is not a medication schedule that can be adjusted, fasting is not a good idea for patients with this type of medication schedule. Further, some heart patients experience shortness of breath, or light-headedness and fasting can exacerbate these symptoms if blood sugar becomes low. As there are many different types of heart conditions, it is necessary to consult a physician before deciding if fasting is right for you.

- **Those with diabetes**

As those with diabetes have struggled with their blood sugar, fasting is likely not a good choice for them. When you fast, your body must find other sources of sugar in order to maintain blood sugar, and in people with diabetes, this can cause complications for their already sensitive blood sugar levels. For people with diabetes, having their blood sugar reach levels that are too high or too low can be very dangerous as their body has a hard time regulating this. Fasting may pose serious health risks for this population.

Side-Effects Associated With Intermittent Fasting

When it comes to side-effects, the number one side-effect of fasting is hunger, as I'm sure you can imagine. As I briefly mentioned though, you may also experience light-headedness and weakness, especially if you are just beginning to add fasting into your diet regime.

There are some side-effects that are to be expected when beginning a fast. These are not necessarily cause for concern, as they are signs of your body adapting to a fast.

Regular side-effects of fasting include:

- Hunger
- Slight dehydration
- Headache
- Irritability
- Lower energy levels
- Constipation
- Lower body temperature

Chapter 5: Intermittent Fasting and Weight Loss

The reason that people choose to fast in order to upregulate autophagy in order to then improve their health is to promote the breakdown of the fat stores in their body. When autophagy is at work, the body will turn to its fat stores for energy by breaking them down. The fat cells that make up the body's fat stores are broken down through the process of autophagy. This can lead to weight loss by way of an induction of autophagy. This is the reason why you have likely heard of fasting as a method for weight loss.

Autophagy and Obesity

While there are many causes of obesity, one of the more recently discovered causes may be related to autophagy or, rather, dysfunction of autophagy within the body. If autophagy is malfunctioning or is under-active in a person's body, this can lead the body to have a much more difficult time using fat stores for energy. This is because of the way the metabolism is affected.

As autophagy becomes improperly regulated, it can lead to a variety of metabolic disorders, obesity being one of them. This can be caused by problems related to autophagy function in fat tissues, especially, which then leads to problems in the breakdown of fat tissues.

For this reason, intermittent fasting is beneficial for fighting obesity in individuals who have problems with autophagy in their bodies. By taking steps to upregulate autophagy by way of intermittent fasting or exercise, this type of individual is able to help their body to use autophagy to its benefit and thus reduce obesity and continue to lose weight.

Calorie Deficit

For all of the methods of intermittent fasting that we went over in chapter three, there is one thing in common between all methods- the foods that you eat when you are not fasting will have a profound impact on your weight loss success or failure in this type of dieting. This is because if you turn to calorie-dense and nutrient-sparse foods in high quantities during your eating hours (or days), you may not end up with a calorie deficit at the end of the week. What this means is that if you are trying IF as a method of weight loss, the basic equation that it comes down to will be;

The number of calories that you ingest - The number of calories you use to survive (for example, walking, eating, breathing) - The extra calories burned from exercise

The number that results from this equation will be either positive or negative. If the number is positive, this means that you ingested more calories than you burned. If the number is negative, this means that you burned more calories than you ingested. If the number is zero, this means that calories ingested and calories burned are equal to one another. If the number is zero, this indicates "breaking even" in terms of your energy. If the number is positive, you can envision it like having more energy than you were able to use. When this occurs, the extra energy is stored as fat in the body. If the number is negative, you used more energy than you had and this translates to weight loss, as once the energy is all used up, the fat stores will begin to be used for additional energy.

This equation explains how bingeing during your eating days or hours can lead to a maintenance of the same weight or even an increase in weight in some cases. If you are using fasting as a means of improved health, then this will be a little different for you, but in general, in order to induce autophagy, you want to achieve a caloric deficit during your times of fasting.

Intermittent Fasting and Metabolism

Metabolism is a large term that describes the breakdown of one thing in order to create energy. In more specific terms, it is all of the processes in the body that work together to maintain life. This happens when you eat food, and it is broken down to create energy for your body to function. This also happens on a smaller level in each cell of the body by way of autophagy as it carries cell components to the lysosome and the breakdown of these cell components is used to create energy for the cell. As we learned earlier, autophagy is initiated by low nutrition levels in the cell and thus, it creates energy for that cell. In this way, it contributes to the overall metabolism of the body by creating energy by way of breaking something down.

When cells are experiencing a lack of nutrition and autophagy is triggered, there is also a release of hormones by the body in an effort to use the energy it is creating in the most efficient way possible. These hormones make the fat stores more easily broken down and more accessible as a source of energy. Because of this, the body's rate of metabolism increases during these times of cellular starvation.

Intermittent Fasting and Energy

The reason that people choose to fast in order to upregulate autophagy in order to then improve their health is to promote the breakdown of the fat stores in their body. The way that the body works when using energy is that it turns to recently-ingested sugars first (like carbohydrates), then it turns to recently stored sugars. If neither of these are available, or once it has used them all up, it will turn to its fat stores for energy by breaking them down. The fat cells that make up the body's fat stores are broken down through the process of autophagy. In this way, if a person can control the energy sources that their body is using, they can control the amount of fat the body is breaking down. This can lead to weight loss by way of an induction of autophagy. This is the reason why you have likely heard of fasting as a method for weight loss. Many people have recently discovered this method of controlling their body's energy sources and have thus been using it as a weight loss technique. While this may seem like something that would not be willingly chosen by a person, it is important to keep in mind that fasting, and starvation are different things. When you fast, your body adjusts itself in order to make the fat stores more accessible for use. This is a response to the starvation that the cells experience, but this can happen without the human themselves experiencing starvation

Weight Loss for Women Over 40

When it comes to the population of women over the age of 40, there are some things that may be different when deciding whether they should be practicing intermittent fasting or not.

Studies show that intermittent fasting can have very beneficial effects for women over the age of 40. Since many women in this age group experience that annoying and persistent belly fat, the study looked at this in particular. In this study, intermittent fasting showed to help women over 40 lose belly fat, which leads to improvements in overall health as well as more satisfaction in terms of physical appearance. By reducing belly fat, women over 40 were able to reduce their risk of metabolic syndrome, which is a disease that has been shown to be especially prevalent in this age group and whose risk is increased with an increase in belly fat. We will look at metabolic syndrome in more detail in chapter seven of this book.

Chapter 6: Intermittent Fasting and Longevity

In this chapter, we will discuss how intermittent fasting can positively affect longevity not only at a cellular level, but on an orgasmic

How Intermittent Fasting and Autophagy Affects Longevity

Autophagy is essential for the longevity of the organism. Autophagy has been shown to have effects on aging and this is why it plays such a large role in longevity. The reason for this is twofold. The first reason is that the cells that it acts in are often damaged or injured and by way of autophagy, the disease or virus that is attempting to infect the organism is unable to spread, allowing the organism to continue living a relatively healthy life. This type of disease control increases the longevity of the organism.

The second reason is that autophagy is essential to maintaining the health of specific tissues and organs, which keeps them running smoothly and functioning at their best, which is also another factor that influences lifespan. If the organs and tissues are healthy, the organism as a whole will be healthy and will keep living.

In these two ways, autophagy plays a large role in the longevity and lifespan of the organisms and their cells.

Quality of Life

While at first autophagy may seem like it has nothing to do with the quality of life, it has many indirect effects on quality of life in general. As you will see in this chapter, autophagy has the possibility to affect the body in many positive and many negative ways. Autophagy can cause diseases and it can also prevent them. It has the possibility to maintain and create the health of the organism and the possibility to also create and maintain disease within the body. Everything in the body comes down to what happens at a cellular level, as it works in a bottom-up way. Whatever happens at the cellular level will work its way up affecting everything at the larger levels before eventually affecting the body as a whole. We will become aware of what is going on at a cellular level once its effects work their way up to our consciousness.

Having a disease, especially one that involves inflammation of some part of the body, can cause high levels of pain and discomfort on a daily basis for the person affected. This affects the quality of life as the person living with pain must take this with them in everything they do.

On the other hand, autophagy can affect the quality of life of a person by maintaining their health and eliminating disease. Inflammation in the short term helps to get rid of diseases, bacterial infections, and any sort of injury. By effectively eliminating disease and injury in a timely manner, the person's quality of life is greatly increased as their health is improved.

When it comes to quality of life, autophagy has been shown to benefit mental health as well. Intermittent fasting which induces autophagy, has been shown to decrease instances of depression and food-related disorders such as binge eating. Its benefits for weight loss also have been shown to improve body image, confidence, and overall self-satisfaction in adults who practice it for one month or more.

In women specifically, who generally have a higher risk of developing depression, intermittent fasting was shown to decrease the levels of depression, anxiety and mood-related disorders such as these. Intermittent fasting leads to an increase in autophagy in the brain, which has many beneficial effects for the individual.

Chapter 7: Intermittent Fasting and Disease

There are numerous benefits that our bodies can gain from intermittent fasting and autophagy. The simplest and most basic way to tell that it is a benefit to our bodies is the fact that it has been preserved by our bodies for this long since the beginning of time. As I mentioned earlier in this book, our bodies are extremely efficient and are designed for survival. If there is something that does not contribute to our survival or our health, our bodies will surely get rid of it or lower its functioning as it can use its precious resources elsewhere for more benefit. Autophagy is still functioning well, and many positive things come of it, which is why it is still an important cell function in multicellular beings to this day.

The main reason why intermittent fasting is so beneficial is that it induces autophagy. Therefore, it is thanks to autophagy that there are so many great things that come from practicing intermittent fasting. We will look at more of the benefits below.

The Immune System

Firstly, we will discuss how beneficial intermittent fasting and therefore, Autophagy is so beneficial for the functioning of the immune system. Autophagy is extremely important for our immune system function. As I briefly mentioned earlier in this book, autophagy plays a part in the immune system by killing infected cells before they can spread and infect other cells. This function of autophagy has perhaps developed over time to adapt to the changes in pathogens that humans are exposed to these days, and it has become quite a benefit to us.

The way that autophagy assists the immune system is similar to the way in which it carries pathogens to the lysosomes to be broken down. When there is a pathogen present, an autophagosome will be created within the cell in just the same way that it is created when there is cell debris and a low level of nutrients within the cell. This pathogen will be engulfed in the autophagosome and will be carried to the lysosome, not for recycling and energy production, but for breakdown and destruction. By this process, which is very similar to the process of energy production, the cell is able to be rid of the pathogens that have infected it without the need for a full immune response, depending on the level of infection in the body. This process that is already occurring in our cells expands its function to serve another purpose which turns out to be greatly beneficial for our general health.

Inflammation

Inflammation is a reaction that occurs in the body in response to things such as pathogens or irritations. Inflammation is a response intended to protect us from whatever signaled the inflammation to occur. It does this by increasing the number of inflammatory cells in the area where the irritant or pathogen is located. The inflammatory cells are there to remove the irritant, promote new cell growth to replace cells that were damaged by the irritant and then to promote overall repair of the area.

Autophagy plays a large role in inflammation as it has a big effect on the inflammatory cells involved. Autophagy has the ability to keep inflammatory cells alive by breaking down old and damaged cell parts and thus keeping the cells healthy and in good working order. It does this in the same way that it keeps any of our other cells working and alive. These inflammatory cells are necessary to keep the organism itself healthy by reaching the site of damage or disease and clearing it out. These inflammatory cells have many jobs to do, and it is important that they stay healthy. Autophagy ensures this and thus has a big impact on the overall health of the organism.

On the outside of the body, inflammation can be identified by redness, swelling, heat to the touch, and pain. This can happen when there is an infection, a physical injury or any other assault to that area.

Inflammation may seem like it is an annoying problem that your body causes you, but it is actually a sign of your body working tirelessly to keep you healthy and remove whatever isn't supposed to be there that is making you sick. We would not be able to heal if it were not for inflammation and autophagy's role in inflammation.

Autophagy also plays a role in reducing inflammation, especially in the brain. Since autophagy has the ability to both keep cells alive and to cause their death, it can control the presence of inflammatory cells and control their exit when the irritant has been removed. By inducing autophagy in your body, you are able to reduce inflammation by having the inflammatory cells be broken down and removed.

Acute Inflammation

There are different types of inflammation. The first one we will discuss is the one you are likely most familiar with, acute inflammation. Acute inflammation has a rapid onset but usually only lasts until the bacteria or the injury is gone. Examples of this include a cut or scrape, tonsillitis, sinusitis, and bronchitis. The inflammatory response occurs at the first sign of infection or virus in the body and these inflammatory cells are no longer present after they have successfully gotten rid of the problem in that area of the body.

Chronic Inflammation

The other type of inflammation is chronic inflammation. Chronic inflammation occurs over a long period of time, from months to years, and has a slower onset than acute inflammation. Acute inflammation can become chronic inflammation if the infection or the injury is not resolved from the initial inflammatory immune response. Chronic inflammation can also occur because of consistent exposure over a long period to a low level of an irritant like allergens or chemicals. When inflammation becomes chronic, we begin to see diseases develop.

Inflammation is beneficial and necessary for proper healing and maintenance of good health, but when it occurs over a long period of time (such as years), this lasting amount of inflammation can actually create problems in the body.

Inflammatory Diseases

"Inflammatory Disease" is an umbrella term for a variety of diseases that involve inflammation in some part of the body, usually over a long period of time. Examples of these diseases include the following;

Allergies

Allergies to something like a cat when you visit someone's house can come about quickly when in the presence of the cat and be gone after a few days once the irritant is removed. Sometimes, however, the inflammation caused by allergies can become chronic and can lead to a condition like hay fever. This is when the nasal pathways become inflamed in an effort to protect the person from inhaling any more of the irritant (like pollen or grass) however, after a few weeks; this inflammation can become quite irritating to the person experiencing it. They will experience things like a stuffed nose which can make it difficult for the person to go about their regular lives. At this point, inflammation that is supposed to help the person becomes more of a burden.

Asthma

Asthma is a disease that is caused by inflammation of the tubes that connect and move air to and from the lungs, as well as the tubes within the lungs. Because these airways are inflamed, they are extra sensitive to everything that the lungs inhale, especially irritants of any sort. When an irritant is inhaled, the already inflamed airways become even more swollen, which makes it very difficult for the person to breathe. Asthma and allergies are closely linked and can act in similar ways or in tandem in the body. Similar to allergies, chronic inflammation can be caused by environmental factors such as pollution in the air or chronic mold exposure.

Inflammatory Bowel Disease

Inflammatory bowel disease is another disease caused by chronic inflammation, and within the term Inflammatory bowel disease (IBD), there are a number of more specific conditions, all characterized by the inflammation of the digestive tract. IBD is caused by an abnormal response in the gut to certain foods, or bacteria and viruses, leading to chronic inflammation.

There are many symptoms that the inflammation of the digestive tract can cause, including nausea, lack of appetite, fever, and fatigue as well as abnormal stools.

One example of an IBD is Crohn's Disease, where any part of the digestive tract can be the site of inflammation. The food that a person puts in their body is very important when they have IBD, as the food will have to go through the digestive tract, and thus the inflamed areas will be involved every time the person ingests food.

All of these inflammatory diseases can come about but can also be improved by the presence of autophagy. Autophagy can keep this inflammation alive, but it can also remedy ·and reduce the occurrence of these diseases if it is induced at the right times by way of intermittent fasting or exercise, as you have learned earlier in this book.

Cancer

Cancer is another umbrella term that includes the entire body. There are numerous types of cancers, but they are all based on the same type of dysfunction of the body's cells. Cancer is caused by malfunctions in the growth of cells, either the uncontrolled growth of new cells or the dramatic slowing of the growth of new cells. Sometimes, this rapid increase in cell creation can cause a tumor, but not all cancers involve tumors. As I mentioned earlier in this book, cell death is a normal part of the body's functioning, and autophagy plays a part in this process. Sometimes, this cell death is not properly executed or communicated and the cells that are meant to die off and be replaced by new ones do not begin the process of cell death. Because of this, there is a large buildup of cells that begin stealing the nutrients and energy from the other cells that were meant to take their place and the body begins to experience impaired immune function as well as other misfunctions.

Cancer cells are able to manipulate autophagy to make it work for them when they need and not when they don't need. Cancer cells use autophagy to their benefit by using the breakdown and energy generation to make energy for themselves to thrive and survive in a nutrient-poor environment. The environment within tumors is nutrient poor because of the large irregular number of cells that must use a regular amount of nutrients. Then, the autophagy is taken advantage of by being used to create nutrients from nothing, by breaking down cell components.

In another way, however, autophagy can actually reduce a person's risk of cancer. This is because of the way that it is able to clear the body of damaged cells. When damaged cells multiply and divide, this can cause a buildup that can become dangerous and eventually cancerous. If autophagy is functioning properly, it should be able to break down these cells before they can build up and, in this way, autophagy keeps a person healthy and cancer-free. It is for this reason that some people choose to take this into their own hands and induce autophagy within their cells. We will look at the ways that people can do this in the next chapter.

How Intermittent Fasting Can Improve Diseases Related to Autophagic Dysfunction

Despite the numerous benefits of autophagy, there are times when it malfunctions or when there is a problem with autophagy in certain areas of the body. This dysfunction can cause diseases and ailments in the people that it impacts. If autophagy is malfunctioning in any way, this can lead to a buildup of debris in the cell, healthy proteins being degraded, cells dying when they are not scheduled to or when they are healthy, and a variety of other issues. When we take steps to upregulate autophagy, by practicing intermittent fasting, you are able to improve the following list of diseases that are caused in large part due to dysfunction of autophagy.

Autoimmune Diseases

Autoimmune diseases are diseases caused by the immune system and inflammation response of the body to begin attacking itself and the tissues of the body that are healthy. This causes the body to damage and destroy its own tissues and cells that are in regular working order, and that would not otherwise be involved in an immune attack. The body confuses unhealthy cells and healthy cells, and this can lead to a variety of diseases depending on where in the body this occurs. There are no known cures for these diseases, and they can only be mediated by symptom-managing treatments.

There are a variety of autoimmune diseases that are common in today's society. We will look at some of them in more depth now.

Autophagy's role in autoimmune diseases is that it keeps the immune cells healthy and strong, but when these cells are not needed, autophagy can end up working against the body as the inflammation becomes painful.

Rheumatoid Arthritis

Rheumatoid arthritis is an example of chronic inflammation that becomes quite painful for the person experiencing it. This is due to the fact that the person is experiencing a self-attack from their immune system as well as chronic inflammation because of this. Chronic inflammation can become quite painful. It can cause a person to feel stiffness and high levels of pain in the affected areas.

Rheumatoid arthritis affects the joints of the body, often in the fingers, wrists, and knees. In this disease specifically, the immune system begins to attack the lining around a joint and this also causes the joint to become inflamed. This inflammation after a long while can also begin to affect the joint's shape and structure as a whole.

Psoriasis

Psoriasis is another autoimmune condition, this time affecting the skin. This autoimmune response causes extra growth of skin, which leads to the dry and scaly appearance of psoriasis. In this condition, the immune system acts as if it is healing a wound on the skin, sending inflammatory cells, and creating many new skin cells. The problem is that there is no wound to heal so the skin ends up being inflamed and the overgrowth of skin cells on top of those that were healthy to begin with can be itchy and painful for the person. The body is unable to discern whether there is a wound or not, leading to the chronic inflammation.

Dementia, Including Alzheimer's Disease

Dementia is a blanket term for a combination of symptoms of cognitive decline, such as forgetfulness and disorientation. Alzheimer's disease is one common example of dementia. One cause of dementia is cell death, which we know by now involves autophagy. This brain cell death happens over a period of time and includes gradual cognitive decline as this happens. The actual causes of dementia including Alzheimer's are not well known, but what is known is that this steady decline is linked to the abnormal cell death.

Autophagy's role in cell death is varied. As we saw earlier, when a cell is damaged or infected beyond repair, autophagy can lead to cell death in order to preserve the health of the organism. In other cases, though the cell death is programmed, and autophagy begins when this programmed cell death is signaled. This is so that new cells can be created to take their place. Sometimes though, as in the case of dementia, cell death occurs similarly to in an autoimmune disorder when it is unprogrammed and unwarranted. When this happens in the brain, the results are quite damaging. This is the opposite of cancer when the programmed cell death malfunctions and the cells that are meant to die do not.

Specific to Women Over 40

Things like blood pressure and cholesterol can lead to severe and life-threatening heart diseases, and fasting has been shown to improve heart health in women. It does this by lowering blood pressure and the "bad" cholesterol, called LDL cholesterol.

Metabolic Syndrome in Women Over 40

By losing belly fat through intermittent fasting and therefore inducing autophagy, women over 40 can reduce their risk of developing metabolic syndrome, which is a disease that encompasses a group of conditions related to high blood pressure and obesity. Metabolic syndrome includes obesity, high cholesterol, high blood sugar, high blood pressure, and a high level of triglycerides which can be harmful to the body. If at least three of these conditions are present in a person, they have metabolic syndrome. This disease is very prevalent in the United States of America and is a growing problem. Intermittent fasting is one of the most effective ways of reducing the risk of developing this disease or even reversing it once a person has it.

Chapter 8: Intermittent Fasting and Hormones

As you know by now, when you fast, your body adjusts itself in order to make its fat stores more accessible for use. This is a response to the starvation that the cells experience, but this can happen without the human themselves experiencing starvation. It does this by adjusting hormone levels. The human body reacts as if it were experiencing starvation at a cellular level to anticipate a possible absence of food. This is yet another example of how our bodies are designed to survive and are built to protect us no matter what the situation. This environment that intermittent fasting creates in the body leads to a release of hormones that have beneficial effects on the body. For example, intermittent fasting in women has been shown to lead to the release of hormones that, in turn, lead to the release of bone minerals such as phosphate and calcium, and the release of these bone minerals leads to increase bone density and strength, which is especially beneficial in women who are over 40, as the risk of developing osteoporosis is very high.

Therefore, inducing autophagy in the body leads to a reduction in the risk of developing osteoporosis in women over 40, and can even lead to improvements in women who have already been diagnosed with it.

Insulin

Intermittent fasting leads to lower levels of insulin active in the blood stream during fasting periods (due to less food, specifically sugars being taken into the body) which then leads to improved use of fat cells for energy which, over time increases the effectiveness of insulin, which is one of the main hormones involved in metabolism, as it signals to cells that there has been an intake in sugar and awakens them to process and store this sugar. By reducing the sugar, the insulin becomes more sensitive to the environment of the body, and over time this is beneficial for the insulin cells and for blood sugar levels of the woman practicing intermittent fasting.

Further, when insulin levels are lower, this leads to the release of another hormone called HGH, which also helps in the breakdown and use of stored fat cells for energy, which leads to weight loss.

Another hormone that is triggered by intermittent fasting is Norepinephrine or Noradrenaline, which becomes released in response to an empty stomach. This hormone encourages the release and the metabolism of fat cells for energy, which also leads to weight loss and improved health due to a reduction in belly fat often found in women over 40.

The Menstrual Cycle

When fasting, some women have experienced changes in their menstrual cycle. The bodies of women are more sensitive to small calorie changes, especially when it comes to a reduction in calorie intake. Since the bodies of women are built to conceive and grow babies, their bodies have to be sensitive to changes in the internal environment to a larger degree than the bodies of men. When the bodies of women experience a reduction in calorie intake, they may have trouble experiencing regular menstrual cycles as the body may deem the internal environment less than ideal for a baby to be grown. This is not to say that women cannot practice IF or fasting of any sort, but that they must keep this in mind when deciding to try a fasting diet.

Poly-Cystic Ovarian Syndrome (PCOS)

PCOS or Polycystic Ovarian Syndrome is something that many women suffer from. This disease leads women's ovaries to develop cysts, which can lead to very painful periods, weight gain and infertility. For women who suffer from Polycystic Ovarian Syndrome, it can be very hard to lose weight. By following intermittent fasting however, women with Polycystic Ovarian Syndrome have been able to lose weight while also having relief from many of the other symptoms associated with it.

It has been shown that a diet high in carbohydrates can negatively affect Polycystic Ovarian Syndrome and can actually exacerbate symptoms. By following an intermittent fasting regime, which is also lower in carbohydrates, women's bodies showed improvement in their general health, reduced the symptoms of this disease (including leading to weight loss), and helped to mitigate the progression of the disease.

Intermittent Fasting and Menopause

When it comes to menopause, many things in your body can feel like they are out of your control. Menopause can lead to weight gain, depression, anxiety, increased risk of heart disease, among others. It will also lead to changes in the hormones and the metabolism of the women that are in menopause, as well as a reduction in the body's sensitivity to insulin.

Because of all of these side-effects of menopause, intermittent fasting can improve these side-effects. Since you know that intermittent fasting leads to an improvement of all of these side-effects, it is a good choice for improving the symptoms of menopause such as weight loss, reducing the risk of heart disease, reducing depression, and so on.

Chapter 9: Exercise and Intermittent Fasting

Exercise functions as a sort of cleanse for the body that doesn't involve restricting food intake to water only. By exercising once per day, you can feel the beneficial effects of exercise on autophagy, and this, when compared to fasting, is much less time-consuming. For best results, a combination of the two will be the most effective for maintaining a healthy weight as well as maintaining good health and reducing the risk of disease overall. With exercise, it is difficult to discern which of its benefits can be attributed to an increase in autophagy and which are from the other bodily functions that exercise induces like an increase in oxygen delivery to your tissues or more efficient functioning of the heart. It is being studied more and more these days; however, in an effort to better understand how much of a role autophagy plays in recovery after exercise.

How Exercise Impacts and Affects Intermittent Fasting

One other way to activate autophagy is through exercise. Aerobic exercise has been shown through studies to increase autophagy in the cells of the muscles, the heart, the brain, lungs, and the liver. When we do aerobic exercise, the heart and lungs work with the muscles to move the body in a specific way (like running or biking). Over time, the heart, lungs and brain will learn to function together more efficiently, which is why exercises get easier the more you do them. Autophagy is upregulated in these specific tissues (heart, lungs, muscles) after aerobic exercise because these are the specific tissues most positively affected by aerobic exercise.

Exercise is the most efficient way to upregulate autophagy as it happens much quicker through aerobic exercise than through starvation. The body is well-equipped to survive, and so fasting takes longer to induce autophagy than exercise does.

Intermittent Fasting and Muscles

When exercising, the muscles and tissues you use will experience small micro-damages, which is what makes them grow back stronger. Think of the way the muscles respond after a workout in the weight room- you are sore for a few days before becoming stronger and growing bigger muscles. This happens in a very similar way at a cellular level. Autophagy comes in when the cells need energy or when they have micro-damages, clearing out the damage and encouraging new cells to take the place of the damaged ones. This leads to growth and regeneration in the specific tissues impacted by specific types of exercise and is one of the many reasons why exercise is so beneficial for the human body.

Remember how we saw in the first chapter of this book, that one of the common myths associated with intermittent fasting is that it could lead to a loss of muscle mass. This is untrue, however, as the body likes to keep its muscle at almost all costs. The body needs muscle and wants us to hold onto it, which comes from the days when humans were hunter-gatherers, so losing muscle is not something that will happen easily, especially not if you are ingesting enough protein and food in general during your eating periods.

As women get older, their muscle mass decreases. For this reason, exercising is great for women of this age in particular because of the increase in muscle mass that it leads to. You will not get bulky if you incorporate some weight or strength training into your exercise routine, it will only help you as it will help to restore some of the muscle mass lost due to age.

How Women Over 40 Can Safely Exercise in Combination With Intermittent Fasting

Keeping your exercise levels to a minimum while fasting is often necessary as your body will not have as much readily-available sugars or carbohydrates to provide you with the quick energy needed for a workout. This is especially important if you are beginning a fasting regimen for the first time. Your body will need time to adjust to fasting without being extra drained from working out as well. If you are planning to increase your levels of autophagy through a combination of fasting and exercise, wait until your body has adapted to your fasting routine before adding in the exercise portion of the plan.

For women more specifically, as I mentioned at the beginning of this chapter, women may experience some different effects when they attempt IF than men do. Because of this, women may want to use exercise as their main method of autophagy induction if they are trying to conceive or if they have experienced irregularities with their menstrual cycle in the past. They can also use a combination of IF and exercise, with shorter periods of IF such as 12 and 12, coupled with an aerobic exercise routine.

One final thing to keep in mind is to ensure that you are not working too hard in terms of exercise on days that you are more heavily fasting, as your body may be feeling more tired than usual as it gets used to the new fasting routine.

Since exercising helps women to regain some of the muscle mass lost due to age, it can be greatly beneficial for women to exercise into their older years. It is important to be aware of how to do this safely though. It can be safer to stick to low-impact exercises, so exercises that avoid jumping or any sort of quick, jarring movements. Instead, spending some time on an exercise bike (or a real bike) or elliptical machine can be good as they reduce impact and are therefore better for a woman's joints. Things like running involve more impact, so if you have joint pain, it is best to avoid this type of exercise. Further, lifting some small weights or walking with weights in your hands can help you to build back some muscle, which will lead to an increase in your resting rate of metabolism (the number of calories your body burns when it is just sitting, at rest in order to execute living functions such as breathing or sitting) which will add to the weight loss effects of intermittent fasting. These two combined are a great positive lifestyle change for women over 40 to consider, as their overall health will be greatly improved by the increase in muscle, the improvement of their joint health and the lowered risk of diseases such as heart disease (which is reduced by doing aerobic exercise and by intermittent fasting). Staying active in your 40's is a great decision, intermittent fasting aside, and every woman who is capable should add exercise into their lives, regardless of the diet that they follow.

Chapter 10: Intermittent Fasting Tips to Increase Success

Before you begin fasting, there are some things that you will want to do to prepare yourself. It may be difficult mentally and physically, especially if you are new to fasting. Your mindset will become very important as you are fasting, especially the longer you fast at one time. Getting yourself into the proper mindset before you begin will help you to stay focused while you are fasting.

Ensure You Are Fasting in a Healthy Way

When it comes to fasting, it is important to ensure that you approach it in a way that will be beneficial for our health, and that will not do more harm than good.

Firstly, you want to maintain flexibility with yourself and your body when fasting. If you are not feeling well as you are trying to fast, don't be afraid to eat a small amount on your fast days. This is especially true at the beginning when you first introduce fasting into your diet. If you try a water fast for example, and you feel lightheaded and weak, you may decide that you want to instead try an intermittent fasting method like 5:2 which would allow you to eat on your fast days, but in a greatly restricted amount. If you have your mind set on a 24-hour water fast, then try the 5:2 method a few times before you try the full water fast in order to get your body comfortable with reduced amounts of food first.

Increase Your Water Intake

As I mentioned, dehydration can accompany fasting since much of our water intake throughout the day comes from the food we eat, like fruits or vegetables. If you are feeling like you are dehydrated while fasting (dry mouth, headache), it is important to increase your water intake. You will also want to ensure you drink enough water each time you fast afterward. The recommendation is about two liters per day, but of course, this depends on your body size. In general, eight glasses of water that are about eight ounces each should give you enough water to be hydrated but when fasting, this must increase to about nine to thirteen glasses. This works out to be between two and three liters of water.

Pay Attention to Your Body

If you are feeling very unwell while you are fasting, it is important to know when to stop fasting. It is normal to feel fatigued, hungry, and maybe irritable when you fast, but you may want to stop your fast if you feel completely unwell. In order to be safe, for your first few times fasting, keep the duration shorter, and work your way up to the desired amount of time. Also, keep some food on you in case you need to eat something due to low blood sugar or feeling unwell. Remember that you are fasting in order to take care of your body and your health and it should not make you feel worse.

Increase Protein Intake

Ensuring that you eat enough protein while fasting will have numerous benefits for you. Protein takes longer to digest, which means that the energy you get from protein will be longer lasting than the energy you get from other sources like carbohydrates- which is used up quite quickly. Eating enough protein will help to keep your hunger at bay, especially if you are doing the 5:2 method or a method where you will eat small amounts on your fasting days. This will keep you from having an energy "crash" similar to a sugar crash after you have quickly used up the sugars you have ingested.

Select The Foods You Eat Wisely

When you do break your fast or when you are eating small amounts on fasting days, choose the foods you eat wisely. You want to properly prepare your body to fast and keep it healthy while you do so. In addition to eating enough protein, you want to make sure that the other foods you eat are real, whole foods. Whole foods are those which are as close to those found in nature as possible. These are things like meats, vegetables, fruits, fish, eggs, and legumes. This will give you all of the nutrients you need to stay healthy. Eating fast food and processed foods on the days that you are not fasting will leave you feeling tired and without energy, especially if you are fasting the next day or have fasted the day before.

Consider Supplementation

Supplementing may be very beneficial and even necessary when fasting to maintain and improve health. Some essential nutrients and minerals that your body would greatly benefit from like Omega-3's or iron may be difficult to get in adequate amounts if you are fasting. For this reason, supplementing them may benefit you in terms of keeping you feeling healthy and energetic, as well as keeping your brain functioning to its full potential. You can take specific nutrients on their own in pill-form or you can opt for a multivitamin that will include all of the most essential vitamins and minerals for overall good health. These vitamins and minerals may differ from those that we looked at in the previous chapter, as those included the vitamins and minerals that are known to induce autophagy. The vitamins included in a multivitamin will be those that are known to promote good overall health and those that are usually obtained through a balanced, whole food diet.

Avoid Over-Doing It in the Beginning

Keeping your exercise levels to a minimum while fasting is often necessary as your body will not have as much readily-available sugars or carbohydrates to provide you with the quick energy needed for a workout. This is especially important if you are beginning a fasting regimen for the first time. Your body will need time to adjust to fasting without being extra drained from working out as well. If you are planning to increase your levels of autophagy through a combination of fasting and exercise, wait until your body has adapted to your fasting routine before adding in the exercise portion of the plan.

When Not to Fast

There are times when fasting is not recommended for a person, no matter how used to fasting they may be. If your fasting day comes around and you are feeling any of the following symptoms, fasting that day will not be advisable for you. Knowing when to decide not to fast is important for your health and wellbeing.

If you are feeling sick, including nausea, diarrhea, and general feelings of sickness, take that day or the next few days off of fasting until you are feeling one hundred percent better. Your body needs all of the nutrition it can get while it is trying to fight off a sickness and fasting will be taxing to the body, which will make it very difficult for it to fight off the illness.

If you are feeling weak to the point of not being able to do normal daily tasks, then fasting is not a good idea. Fasting can leave you feeling more tired and having less mental clarity, so doing so when you already feel extreme fatigue will only make this worse. Eating a regular and balanced day's worth of food will have many more benefits for your body than fasting in this case.

If you are feeling faint for any reason, do not begin your fast. If you have already begun your fast, break it and ingest some type of food as you may be experiencing very low blood sugar. If you are feeling faint, putting your body into ketosis and having to use up all of its sugar stores is not a good idea and can be dangerous to you.

Things to Take Note of to Ensure Success

Before you begin to fast, as with anything else you set out to do in life, it is important to be aware of your objectives and your motivations for doing it in the first place. It is unlikely that you are doing anything in life without a reason or a motivation for doing so, and if you think you are then maybe your objective is there in the back of your mind somewhere. Think about your objective before you begin, because when you are in the middle of your fast, you will need to look to that objective or motivation to keep you from changing your mind right then and there and breaking your fast for a doughnut.

The Biggest Obstacle: Your Mind

Everybody's objective will differ slightly and will likely be quite personal to them. Maybe you want to reduce your risk of cancer because it runs in your family. Maybe you have been obese for the majority of your life, and you are trying this as a means of weight loss and health improvement. Maybe you heard about it and challenged yourself to try it for a few months to see how it feels. Whatever your objective, writing it down will help to solidify it and make it real. Then, when you are wondering why on earth you decided to put yourself through this on the first day of your fast, you can look at that objective that you wrote down and it will re-inspire you to continue. When it comes to mindset, being aware of your motivation is extremely beneficial.

When it comes to something like fasting, the mental game is the biggest part of it. You already know that your body can survive without ingesting food for the time that you plan to fast. You know that you will be giving it food at the end of this fasting period. You know that your body will likely even be better for having fasted. What all this means is that the part that makes it very difficult is the mental part. During a fast, the mindset will play a huge part in how you feel.

What you choose to focus on during your fast will determine if you are having a terrible time and counting down the hours until you can eat again, or if you barely notice them going by. By focusing on what you are depriving yourself of, you will see everything as a punishment you are putting yourself through. This will make it very difficult for you to make it through your fasting period as everything except water and coffee will seem like it has been placed before your eyes to punish you. By instead looking at the things that you are giving yourself- like tea, black coffee and water and appreciating these things, it will help you to rediscover how refreshing and nourishing water is, a fact that we take for granted in places where our water is clean and drinkable. You will be able to taste the coffee beans without the cream and sugar that cover up their beauty. You will be able to appreciate the tea leaves that spend time growing in order to end up in this cup of yours. You will also appreciate your food that much more when you reach your eating window and you can eat whatever you want. By viewing your day through the lens of appreciation instead of deprivation, you will have a much easier time with your fast.

Your Expectations

By expecting that there will be some uncomfortable side-effects like hunger and irritability, you can greet them with the feeling of "Oh hello, I have been expecting you." Rather than "Oh no I am feeling so terrible what is going on?" If you are not surprised that you will feel a little bit uncomfortable while your body adapts to your fast, you will be able to greet it rather than fight it, which will make you much more comfortable with it all.

It is important to recognize when fasting that this is a choice you are making for your health, your body or whatever specific objective you have. You must recognize that this is a choice you are consciously making and that you have decided to go through these times of fasting in order to later receive the benefits. If you lose sight of the fact that this is a choice you are making, you may begin to feel like a victim or like the universe is punishing you. This victim mindset will only make things harder for you. By taking responsibility for your decision to fast, you will not allow yourself to slip into this negative mindset and will instead feel confident and in control of your decision. This will help you to view things through the lens of appreciation rather than deprivation like I outlined above.

Your Emotions While Fasting

You can prepare as much as you like, but while you are fasting, you could meet some unexpected feelings. Challenging your body and mind often brings up many feelings for us, as it puts us in a state of self-reflection and deep thought. This is normal. Think about if you decided to run a marathon. While running, as your legs desperately want to give up and your body is tired, your mind will likely go to some deep places that they do not go when you are going about your regular daily duties. Fasting is similar to the marathon in this way as it can be very challenging for both the body and the mind.

When emotions come up during your fast, it is important to know what to do with them. The first step is to acknowledge them. By acknowledging these emotions, you can tap into them and examine them in more depth. The next step is to write them down. This can be a very quick note of how you are feeling or what is the most challenging part for you. By writing it down, you are processing this emotion and you are able to address it instead of pushing it away. When we push our emotions away, they do not really go away; they just go dormant for a short period of time only to come up later. By addressing them, you can examine what is going on inside of you.

An example of this is if you begin fasting as a means of losing weight. On your first day, you are struggling with hunger and cravings and you begin to feel like you might fail. You begin to fear failing and what this would mean for your weight and your body image. You begin to feel sad because you are so uncomfortable with your body. This spiral of emotions is normal. If you just tried to push these emotions away every time they came up, you would keep feeling them over and over until one day you cracked and decided to break your fast, never to attempt it again. By pushing away our strongest feelings, we risk them coming back so strongly that they send us right back to where we came from.

As you begin fasting, keep a small journal with you so that you can write down notes about how you are feeling. Even if you don't have the time to examine your feelings deeply, write them down so that you can come back to them later in order to look into them more deeply.

How to Maintain a Specific Mental State While Fasting

During your fast is when your planning is put to the test. This section includes some tips to keep in mind to help you maintain your ideal fasting mindset throughout your entire fast.

Using Healthy Distractions

It can be easy to plan the mindset that you want to go into your fast having, but while you are fasting, this may be difficult to maintain. It becomes more difficult in practice when you are faced with the reality of the challenge, rather than just the idea of it. One way to help yourself, especially in the beginning of your fasting, is to distract yourself healthily. If you are at work throughout the day, this work may distract you from the fact that you are fasting. When not busy, many people tend to eat out of boredom and while fasting, this urge to eat when not truly hungry will only serve to remind you of the fact that you are not eating. By keeping your mind occupied, you are able to pass the time in other ways that don't have to include eating. Examples of healthy distractions include; going for a walk, watching a movie, playing a game or a sport (lightly), visiting friends, working on a hobby. Any of these can keep your mind occupied and your body busy so that the urge to eat doesn't come about from boredom alone and make it more difficult than it needs to be to fast.

Exploring Your Emotions

As we discussed in the previous section, if you are examining your emotions while fasting and looking deep into them in order to get closure within yourself, you will be more likely to succeed when fasting. It is easy to get off track if you are approaching your fast with the mindset that you need to force yourself into this new way of life. By trying to force yourself, you may just end up feeling resentment and later bingeing when you are meant to be fasting. Because of this, it is important to be able to maintain your positive mindset while fasting. At the end of each day, go back to your notebook, where you wrote down your emotions throughout the day. While you are doing this, spend some time to look more deeply into the emotions that have come up for you, by writing down what you feel as you explore these feelings internally. By spending some time to do this at the end of a fasting day, you can begin the next fasting day fresh without bringing anything forward.

As we discussed in the previous section, being able to look at your fast as something that is completely within your control, that you are consciously deciding to do is important when trying to maintain the perspective of appreciation and gratitude for what you are able to drink while fasting and what you are able to eat when your fast is over.

Why Setting Clear Guidelines to Follow Post-Fast is Important

Research has shown that how and when you break your fast is actually just as important as the fast itself. This part of the fast is known as the *refeeding* phase. Because this part of the fast is just as important as the fast itself, ensuring that you have clear guidelines set out for yourself about how you will break your fast is necessary. This will ensure that you can do so in the best way possible, as it may be difficult to think through this type of process with a clear mind after you have just finished fasting for hours. Ensuring that the guidelines are already set out for you will ensure your success post-fast.

If you were to allow yourself to eat whatever you wanted to after your fast, you would likely go straight to the foods that you had been craving all day, and the chances of these being vegetables and lean protein are quite slim. By not setting any guidelines for yourself, you may begin to decide that you need to "reward" yourself at the end of your fast by letting yourself eat anything you like in any amount you like. If there are no guidelines to follow, there is no place to stop, and you may end up in a bingeing cycle of eating too much and then eating nothing- and so on. Aside from being unhealthy for you and possibly reversing the progress you made by fasting, this would lead to uncomfortable indigestion and an unhappy gut for you.

Another reason why setting clear guidelines is important for breaking your fast is because the foods that you turn to in moments of intense hunger and cravings are usually carbohydrate and calorie-rich foods that do not keep you full for very long. These foods usually do not contain protein which is the longest lasting source of energy. Vegetables are also low in calories but high in volume so they are another good option to ensure you feel satiated and energized without having painful indigestion and a lack of energy.

How to set Clear Guidelines for Yourself Post-Fast

Meal planning is extremely beneficial for any sort of diet, as combatting cravings and hunger is often a large part of dieting. Since you know beforehand that you will be dealing with the mental struggles associated with these cravings, it is important to set yourself up for success by taking all decision-making and preparation work out of the equation post-fast. If you were to leave it up to your post-fast self to decide what to eat for dinner, to grocery shop for it, and to prepare it, the chances of this post-fast self saying "Whatever, I'm too hungry" and ordering a pizza instead are quite high. By having your post-fast meal already portioned and prepared, only needing to be microwaved, you will allow yourself to break your fast in the way you planned without giving yourself the time or space to decide to break fast in any other way. By making it easier for yourself to microwave a pre-planned meal than to order and wait for a pizza, you know exactly which option you will choose every time.

Another way to set clear guidelines for yourself is to make sure that the foods you know you will crave and reach for will not be easily accessible. If you know that you crave chips and salty snacks, and that as soon as you break your fast, you will turn to those, keep those out of the house so that you are unable to eat them even if you wanted to. Keeping only the foods, you plan to break your fast with within reach will make it so that you will have no choice but to eat the foods you planned to.

How to Properly and Carefully Break Your Fast

How you break, your fast will depend on the time of day at which it occurs and the type of fast that you participated in. In this section, I will go over some general rules fort breaking your fast, but keep in mind that you will need to adjust these slightly to fit your personal fast. The important things to keep in mind are the same among all fasts however.

Breaking your fast is all about showing your body that you are not undergoing starvation and that there is not going to be an ongoing lack of food, but that it is going to have to get used to eating less often than it used to. After some time, it will adjust to this, but in the beginning, it will be attempting to keep you alive as it thinks that there has been some type of food drought.

There are specific times when it is most important to break your fast in a very deliberate way. These times are closer to the beginning of your introduction of fasting, when you change the duration of fasting if you are working your way up to longer fasts and when you fast for the first time in a while. While it is always important to break your fast with clear guidelines, at these times, it is most important as the chances of experiencing some stomach upset post-fast are the highest. Follow the guidelines below to see what things you should be keeping in mind when you break your fast.

Start With Water

If you are breaking fast in the morning, begin by drinking a glass of water before anything else. This will put something into your stomach and tell your body that it is time to begin working for the day. If you are breaking fast in the evening and have been drinking water all day, stick to water with your meal as you don't want to feed your digestive system too much at once.

Insulin Sensitivity and Carbohydrates

Remember in chapter four how we discussed circadian rhythms, the sleep-wake cycle and how this coincides with specific times of the day? This actually has a lot to do with how and when we should break fast as well. It has been shown that there is a circadian rhythm of metabolism (the body's use of chemical processes to create energy) that is closely linked to the circadian rhythm of the sleep and wake cycle. The metabolic circadian rhythm is so closely linked to the sleep-wake cycle that the quality of sleep that you get can impact the body's ability to use insulin effectively. There are certain times within this circadian rhythm of metabolism where the body is better able to use insulin to regulate blood sugar and energy levels than other times. When breaking fast, you want to be aware of this cycle and break your fast along with the body's ability to most effectively use insulin. Insulin is what regulates blood sugar by responding to sugar levels in the blood and opening or closing channels through which sugar molecules travel into and out of cells.

Because of the cycle of insulin sensitivity, it is better to break your fast with a low-carbohydrate meal so that your blood sugar levels to not spike too high. Because of the lack of food that has been ingested, the blood sugar levels will have been regulated based on this. If this suddenly changes with a high-carb meal, this can shock the body's insulin system causing it to suddenly need to work on overdrive in order to regulate the spike in blood sugar that the body has just experienced.

Avoid Known Digestive Irritants

When you break your fast, you want to do so with foods that will be easily digested, as your digestive system was essentially sleeping while you were fasting. If there are any foods that you know are difficult for you to digest, or that you know tend to irritate your stomach or your digestive system in general, you want to avoid these foods. While your digestive system may already be having some trouble waking up fully, you don't want to give it any more stress by ingesting foods that will be difficult for it to deal with. This will also save you some uncomfortability during digestion. While you likely have some foods that you know personally bother you, the following foods are ones that should be avoided post-fast in general as they tend to be difficult to digest.

- Nuts
- Seeds
- Dairy
- Alcohol
- Eggs
- Red Meat
- Nut butters
- Seed butters

After your first meal or two, you should have no problem with these foods if you normally digest them just fine. If you eat them at your second meal and have some trouble digesting them, try waiting a little longer next time before you reintroduce them.

Break Fast Slowly

While eating your first meal, you will likely feel the urge to eat very quickly and consume as much as you can as quickly as you can as it has been a while since you last ate. It is important to resist this urge as you may experience some bloating or uncomfortably in the digestion of your food.

Practice mindfulness while eating. This means taking every bite slowly and ensuring that you taste and chew each bite fully. Notice how the food feels in your mouth and how it tastes. Remain in the present moment, focused on the bite you are taking and try not to think of anything else. Since you have not eaten in a while, try to enjoy the first meal you have after you fast. Instead of eating it so quickly that you don't even remember the taste of it, take your time to savor it.

Do Not Overeat

It is important when you break your fast that you do not overeat. Since your digestive system has been resting during your fast, giving it too much work to do all at once can lead to indigestion and difficulty digesting the amount of food that it has been fed, which can lead to uncomfortable side-effects for you.

As you learned previously, mindful eating will come in handy again here. Practicing this type of eating will help you to not only enjoy the food and appreciate it, but it will help you to eat slowly. By taking your time with each bite and ensuring that you chew it and taste it, eating slower will happen naturally. Further, as you learned earlier in this chapter, meal planning- especially portion planning, is another way to ensure you do not overeat when you break your fast.

The Eating Window

After your first meal, there will be a window of time in which you are going to eat your meals before fasting again. During this window, you can eat as often or as little as you like. Be aware that you want to begin setting yourself up for your next fast near the end of your eating window, so eating your last meal right before the end of this window is advised.

You can treat this window however you like eating two meals or four for example. How you decide to eat in your eating window will also depend on the way that you have split your fasting and eating- whether over days of the week or hours of the day. This is the part of fasting with the most flexibility, so feel free to experiment with your meals here in order to see what works the best for your body.

Things to Watch Out for

If you do decide that fasting is right for you, there may be a time during your fast that you must seek medical advice. Knowing when to seek medical advice and when you may be dealing with regular side-effects of fasting is important to ensure you are fasting in a healthy manner.

Side-effects that signal for you to consult a doctor

- Nausea
- Dizziness
- Bloody stools
- Vomiting
- Loss of consciousness
- Abdominal or chest pain

If you experience any of the above symptoms while fasting, consult a doctor as there may be some complications or other problems that fasting has brought about.

If you experience diarrhea, this may be caused by a number of things, but more importantly, diarrhea can lead to other more serious issues like dehydration, dizziness, cramping and malnutrition. If you experience diarrhea while fasting, you can end your fast and see if this clears up though home methods such as hydrating, restoring electrolytes and consuming potassium-rich foods. If it does, consider trying a different kind of fast or visiting your doctor to determine other, safer ways to fast. However, if you are experiencing severe diarrhea along with any pains or severe dehydration, contact a doctor immediately.

Chapter 11: Intermittent Fasting for Women Over 40

Since this book is focused on intermittent fasting for women over the age of 40, we are going to take the final chapter of this book to discuss how intermittent fasting may be different and some of the unique challenges that can come along with this if you are a woman over the age of 40. There are already differences between the ways in which intermittent fasting affects men and women, so adding the difference in age makes things a little more complicated yet. Many studies related to diets and weight loss are focused on men in and around the 30 years old range. Luckily though, there are studies and resources out there for women over 40, and here I have brought them together for you to get all of the information you will need to make a safe and informed decision for your health and your body.

How Intermittent Fasting Will Affect Women Over 40 Differently

There are some diseases or health-related issues that are more prevalent in women over 40, and in this section, we will look at these and how they are affected by intermittent fasting and inducing autophagy.

Some of the diseases or health-related issues that are more likely to affect women over the age of 40 include joint pain, arthritis, lower metabolism (which can lead to weight gain), reduced muscle mass, sleep disturbances, increased levels of belly fat, osteoporosis and other common but weight and age-related diseases such as heart disease or diabetes. By practicing intermittent fasting and losing weight; as a result, you will reduce your risk of developing several of these diseases. By inducing autophagy, you are reducing your risk of those diseases that are not as closely related to weight, such as cancer and heart attacks.

Joint Health

In women over 40, there is much more risk of developing joint issues such as knee pain, wrist, elbow, or shoulder pain. This is due to an increase in age and more risk of arthritis or low back and other joint pain due to age and overuse. In studies where women over 40 practiced intermittent fasting for a period of time, they were found to have decreased levels of joint pain, arthritic symptoms, and low back pain.

How Women Over 40 Can Benefit From Intermittent Fasting

As you have seen evidenced throughout this book, intermittent fasting is extremely beneficial for women over 40, and most of the research done around this type of diet regime points to positive effects. It is quite difficult to find research that doesn't support intermittent fasting for women over 40 as an effective tool for weight loss, improved health, and better overall mental health. As long as intermittent fasting is followed in a safe manner, the results can be extremely positive!

Things for Women Over 40 to Keep in Mind

Supplementing may be very beneficial and even necessary when fasting to maintain and improve health. Some essential nutrients and minerals that your body would greatly benefit from like Omega-3's or iron may be difficult to get in adequate amounts if you are fasting. For this reason, supplementing them may benefit you in terms of keeping you feeling healthy and energetic, as well as keeping your brain functioning to its full potential. You can take specific nutrients on their own in pill-form or you can opt for a multivitamin that will include all of the most essential vitamins and minerals for overall good health. These vitamins and minerals may differ from those that we looked at in the previous chapter, as those included the vitamins and minerals that are known to induce autophagy. The vitamins included in a multivitamin will be those that are known to promote good overall health and those that are usually obtained through a balanced, whole food diet.

Nutrients You Need and How to Get Them

In this section, we are going to look at the most beneficial nutrients for your body and where/ how you can find them when following a specific diet. For women over the age of 40, it is important to ensure that you are getting all of the nutrients that your body needs, especially if you are trying to lose weight or are following a regime that includes fasting. To ensure that during your fasting periods, you are as healthy as possible, supplementation is something that could be considered, to ensure that you are feeding your body the nutrients it needs. It is always preferable to get the nutrients you need from whole foods rather than from supplements, but in some cases, when you cannot get everything you need from the foods in your diet alone (especially if you are eating less calories), then supplementation is always better than nothing. Below, we will look at some whole food sources as well as some supplements that you may wish to consider.

Omega 3 Fatty Acids

These are something that are essential since they cannot be made in our bodies. Omega-3 Fatty Acids are substances that are necessary to get from your diet as the body cannot make them on its own. These fatty acids are a certain type in a list of other fatty acids, but this type (Omega-3) are the most essential and the most beneficial for our brains and bodies in general. They have numerous effects on the brain including reducing inflammation (which reduces the risk of Alzheimer's) and maintaining and improving mood and cognitive function, including memory. Omega-3's have these greatly beneficial effects because of the way that they act in the brain, which is what makes them so essential to our diets. Omega-3 Fatty Acids increase the production of new nerve cells in the brain by acting specifically on the nerve stem cells within the brain, causing new and healthy nerve cells to be generated.

Omega-3 fatty acids can be found in fish like salmon, sardines, black cod, and herring. It can also be taken as a pill-form supplement for those who do not eat fish or cannot eat enough of it. It can also be taken in the form of a fish oil supplement like krill oil.

Omega-3's are by far the most important nutrient that you need to ensure you are ingesting because of the numerous benefits that come from it, both in the brain and in the rest of the body. While supplements are often a last step when it comes to trying to include something in your diet, for Omega-3's the benefits are too great to potentially miss by trying to receive all of it from your diet.

Sulphoraphane

Brussels Sprouts, Cabbage, Kale, Broccoli Sprouts have in common? All of these green vegetables have one thing in common- they all contain Sulforaphane. Sulforaphane is a plant chemical that is found naturally in these vegetables. This is an antioxidant that acts in a similar way to turmeric and thus has similar benefits. Sulforaphane like turmeric, induces autophagy in the brain which helps to reduce the risk of Alzheimer's, Parkinson's and dementia which are all neurodegenerative diseases. *Neurodegenerative* means that the cells in the brain called nerves are damaged and broken down, which leads to cognitive decline like Alzheimer's or physical decline as in Parkinson's. These vegetables can help to treat these diseases by slowing their progression, as they are all diseases that come about over time. There is no cure yet, but the treatment at this stage involves delaying the progression of these diseases.

Sulforaphane can be found in the aforementioned vegetables, but the strongest source is in broccoli sprouts. It can also be taken concentrated in a supplement form.

Calcium

Calcium is beneficial for the healthy circulation of blood, and for maintaining strong bones and teeth. Calcium can come from dairy products like milk, yogurt, and cheese. It can also be found in leafy greens like kale and broccoli and sardines.

Magnesium

Magnesium is beneficial for your diet, as it also helps you to maintain strong bones and teeth. Magnesium and Calcium are most effective when ingested together, as Magnesium helps in the absorption of calcium. It also helps to reduce migraines and is great for calmness and relieving anxiety. Magnesium can be found in leafy green vegetables like kale and spinach, as well as fruits like bananas and raspberries, legumes like beans and chickpeas, vegetables like peas, cabbage, green beans, asparagus and brussels sprouts, and fish like tuna and salmon.

Exogenous Ketones

When tested on animal models, even when they were ingested on a normal carbohydrate intake diet, these exogenous ketones proved to be beneficial in terms of helping the models with problems like seizures, being anti-cancer, anti-inflammation, and anti-anxiety, which are the diseases that we normally see to be assisted by ketosis (which is the state the body enters when it is using fat as a source of fuel instead of carbohydrates), just like we saw in the first few chapters of this book.

Electrolytes

When you first begin following an intermittent fasting regime, having Electrolyte depletion is quite common. This is because of water weight loss through fat and a lower carbohydrate intake, which is often common, as we have discussed. By taking electrolyte supplements, this can help to avoid a deficiency in common electrolytes, like magnesium, potassium and sodium. This is also why you should ensure you are getting enough dietary sodium, as this is an electrolyte that you need. Along with this, though, you will need to ensure you are drinking enough water to avoid dehydration.

Iron

This one is a little tricky, but it is worth noting. Iron should be obtained in the right amounts in your diet through whole foods. If you feel like you might be deficient in iron and you are having trouble getting it in the foods you eat, you can visit your doctor for advice on this topic. Iron cannot be supplemented without being referred by a doctor first, as it is something that they would like you to first try to get from your food. If this is becoming a problem, they can give you supplements to take. This is especially a concern if you are not eating much red meat, and this may lead your doctor to want you to begin supplementing. Make an appointment with your doctor to find out more about this topic.

Vitamin D

Vitamin D is found in some foods that have been fortified with it, but in a natural sense, it can be found in only a few foods. These include cheese, fatty fish like salmon and tuna as well as egg yolks. Another source is mushrooms that have been exposed to UV rays, so the organic ones are likely of this sort.

Vitamin D can be absorbed naturally through sun exposure, so if you live in a sunny place, make sure you get our for some walks or some timer with the sun on your skin. If you live in a colder or more gloomy place, consider purchasing a lamp that mimics the sun and provides you with vitamin D in your house. On a sunny day, even if it is cold going outside and getting sun on your face will give you vitamin D.

This one is something that everyone should be conscious of, but it is especially necessary to examine if you are following a specific diet.

Bioactive Compounds

Bioactive compounds are compounds found within foods that act in the body in beneficial ways. The bioactive compounds found within berries, such as Acai Berries, Strawberries, and Blueberries are very beneficial for your health. The bioactive compounds in these specific types of berries work in the brain to induce autophagy and reduce inflammation. This leads to the protection of brain cells in this case from *oxidative stress*. Oxidative stress is something that can happen within the brain when there is an imbalance of oxygen, which can cause reduced cognitive functioning. These berries and their induction of autophagy helps to reduce this by keeping the balance of oxygen at a healthy level.

Conclusion

In anything new that we try, there is a chance that we may fall off track. Fasting or following a new diet plan are no different. The focus should not be on the fact that you fell off but on how you decide to come back and approach it again. You need not give up altogether if you have a day or two where you did not accomplish your full fast. You just need to re-examine your plan and approach it in a different way. Maybe your fasting period was too long for your first try. Maybe your fasting and eating windows did not match up with your sleep-wake cycle as well as they could have. Any of these factors can be adjusted to better suit your lifestyle needs and make fasting or a specific diet work for you. As I mentioned earlier in this book, being able to be flexible with yourself is something that trying a new diet regimen like this can teach you. With the human body, there is never a right or a wrong way to approach anything; there is only a multitude of different ways and some that will be better for your specific body and mind than others. Being open to trying different variations and adjusting your plan as you go can be the difference between success and deciding to give up.

If you fall off track, scale your plan back a little bit and try it again. If you are worried that you are not doing enough, begin with the scaled back plan, and get used to this first, you can always increase your fasting times later on once you know you are completely comfortable with a shorter fasting time.

If this book has taught you anything, the hope is that it has taught you how many variables are involved when it comes to health and wellness. This book aimed to share with you the plethora of options that are available to you when it comes to autophagy and inducing it within the cells of your body.

Think back on the many options that were laid out for you in this book involving diet options and specific foods that have the ability to induce autophagy in the brain. It is your job now to decide which of these foods or supplements to include in your life and to practice a sort of trial and error, noting which ones make you feel great and which ones you prefer to go without. With all of this information, you can decide which ways fit best with your specific lifestyle and your preferences.

As you take all of this information forth with you, it may seem overwhelming to begin applying this into your own life. Remember, life is a process, and you do not need to expect perfection from yourself. By taking the steps to read this book, you are already on your way to changing your life. IF you fall off of the diet and you need inspiration, come back to the first chapters of this book and remind yourself why you wanted to begin it in the first place.

CPSIA information can be obtained
at www.ICGtesting.com
Printed in the USA
BVHW071456290421
606135BV00001B/69

9 781801 445238